THE
Bodywise
Woman

Second Edition

Judy Mahle Lutter, MA
Lynn Jaffee
Melpomene Institute for Women's Health Research

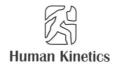

Human Kinetics

Library of Congress Cataloging-in-Publication Data

Lutter, Judy Mahle, 1939-
    The bodywise woman / Judy Mahle Lutter, Lynn Jaffee. -- 2nd ed.
      p. cm.
    Rev. ed. of: The bodywise woman. 1990.
    Includes bibliographical references and index.
    ISBN 0-87322-606-2
    1. Exercise for women.   2. Physical fitness for women.   3. Women-
   -Health and hygiene.   I. Jaffee, Lynn, 1954-   II. Title.
    RA781.B64   1996   96-13088
    613.7'045--dc20   CIP

ISBN: 0-87322-606-2

Acquisitions Editor: Kenneth Mange; **Developmental Editor:** Christine Drews; **Assistant Editor:** John Wentworth; **Editorial Assistant:** Jennifer J. Hemphill; **Copyeditor:** Regina Wells; **Proofreader:** Barbara Erin Cler; **Indexer:** Mary Prottsman; **Graphic Artist:** Yvonne Winsor; **Text Designer:** Judy Henderson; **Photo Editor:** Boyd LaFoon; **Cover Designer:** Jack Davis; **Photographer (cover):** H. Armstrong Roberts/D. Graham; **Illustrators:** Dianna Porter and Studio 2-D; **Printer:** United Graphics

Human Kinetics books are available at special discounts for bulk purchase. Special editions or book excerpts can also be created to specification. For details, contact the Special Sales Manager at Human Kinetics.

Printed in the United States of America   10 9 8 7 6 5 4 3 2 1

Human Kinetics
Web site: http//www.humankinetics.com/

United States: Human Kinetics
P.O. Box 5076
Champaign, IL 61825-5076
1-800-747-4457
e-mail: humank@hkusa.com

Canada: Human Kinetics, Box 24040
Windsor, ON N8Y 4Y9
1-800-465-7301 (in Canada only)
e-mail: humank@hkcanada.com

Europe: Human Kinetics, P.O. Box IW14
Leeds LS16 6TR, United Kingdom
(44) 1132 781708
e-mail: humank@hkeurope.com

Australia: Human Kinetics
57A Price Avenue
Lower Mitcham, South Australia 5062
(08) 277 1555
e-mail: humank@hkaustralia.com

New Zealand: Human Kinetics
P.O. Box 105-231, Auckland 1
(09) 523 3462
e-mail: humank@hknewz.com

Contents

Acknowledgments

Thank you to the additional contributors to this book: Hanna Cooper, Lisa Oswald, Sharon Saydah, Anne Snyder, and Sandra Turbes.

Many other people have helped make this second edition of *The Bodywise Woman* possible. Our thanks to the following:

Martha Stoll Albertson
Barbara Andersen
Bev Anderson
Susie Bergeron
Dr. Martin E. Block
Boeckmann Library at Ramsey
    County Medical Society/
    United Hospital
Boston Women's Health Book
    Collective
Michonne Bertrand
Linda Bunker
Margie Burchell
Linda Camp
Teri Christensen
Nancy Clark
Susan Cushman
Holly Ellison
Meg Ferguson
Robyn Hanscom
Jill Hartnett
Institute for Study of Youth
    Sports at Michigan State
    University
Ruthann Kallenberg
Sarah Keup
Patty Kohls

Pat Kulpa
Chris Kwong
Jessica Larsen
Paula Lawrence
Pat Lyons
Hap Lutter
Melpomene Institute Members
    and Study Participants
Melpomene Staff:
    Mary Lou Carlson
    Eleanor Challen
    Sally Ehlinger
    Linda Feltes
    Karen Larkin
    Gloria Massey
    Judy Remington
    Kendra Young
    Jenna Zark
Stephanie Phillips
Sharon Simpson
Eva Sipkins
Karin Soli
Angela Tucker
Vancouver Women's Health
    Collective
Pam Van Zyl York
Megan Webster

Portraits of Pearl Jackson, Gayle Winegar, and Renell Pettinelli were adapted from profiles that originally appeared in *The Melpomene Journal*, authored by Becky Coleman, Linda Klein, and Janet Tripp.

Thank you to those who helped write the first edition of *The Bodywise Woman:* Janine Benyus, Vicki Novak Johnson, Cynthia Jones, Valerie Lee, and Lee Zurek.

Foreword

I can barely remember a time without sport. I was only three when my father first took me into the San Diego surf, but I can still recall the excitement of running through the hot sand and the thrill of diving for the ocean floor just in time to avoid a huge, frigid wave. When I was seven, I joined my brother's Little League baseball team as a bat girl (at that time, girls weren't allowed to play!). I spent all my allowance on bubble gum and used it to bribe my way into the dugout, just so I could be that much closer to the game. I loved it, but in the end, I just couldn't take sitting on the bench during game after game, wondering what it would be like to just once get to bat, hit the ball, run the bases, make a catch, and celebrate a victory that I'd been a part of creating. At the end of the season, I did what so many frustrated girls in the 1950s must have done when confronted with the male world of sports: I quit.

Luckily, the next summer I found swimming and fell in love again. Through years of training, supportive parents, and dedicated coaches, I was eventually able to achieve what few girls at that time were given a chance to attempt: In 1960, I participated in my first Olympics.

Not every woman who becomes involved in physical activity goes on to win gold medals, but girls and women who participate in sports do have higher levels of confidence, stronger self-images, and lower levels of depression. High school girls who participate in sports have higher body image and self-esteem and are more likely to graduate with better grades. Older women who exercise put themselves at a lower risk of osteoporosis: This is especially important given that 40 percent of all women will have at least one spinal fracture by the time they reach age 80. These days, more and more women are becoming aware of their bodies. Federal legislation such as Title IX and the Amateur Sports Act, both of which I fought hard for, has begun to level the playing field for women of all ages.

The two most important things that my early and continued involvement in swimming gave me weren't gold medals or the fleeting glory that comes with winning, but increased self-esteem and an acute sense of my body. These two gifts have come into play again and again in my life. As a mother of two children, working in network television, and balancing an impossible schedule (as all mothers do), I don't know where I'd be if athletics hadn't taught me to set goals and believe in my ability to see them through—to trust my vision, whether that be winning the 400-meter medley, founding the Women's Sports Foundation, or just getting dinner on the table!

Judy Mahle Lutter, Lynn Jaffee, and the staff of the Melpomene Institute understand implicitly the importance of such gifts. They work tirelessly to share with women everywhere the excitement of being physically active and in touch with your body. They've given us answers to questions about ourselves that our mothers and grandmothers would never have thought to ask. Not being satisfied with that, they continue to seek out new questions and answer them, too, before *we* even think to ask them. These answers are packed into this second edition of *The Bodywise Woman*. Whether you're a seasoned athlete or just beginning to discover your body abilities, Judy Mahle Lutter and Lynn Jaffee have put together a valuable resource to help you become more fit, more confident, and more aware of your potential.

Donna de Varona
Olympic gold medalist swimmer

Preface

Ever wonder how to incorporate physical activity into an already busy schedule, improve your body image, or simply get started on an exercise program? Maybe you've groped with more serious subjects like why your period changes with exercise, what types of physical activity are safe when you are pregnant, or how exercise affects the aging process and vice-versa. If so, this book is for you. In *The Bodywise Woman,* we have taken the best of research and women's personal experiences and combined them to present practical, scientifically sound advice for the woman who is physically active or who wishes to be so.

This second edition of *The Bodywise Woman* is much changed from the first edition: The content has been revised and broadened in light of new research conducted over the last 5 years. Our goal is to provide our readers with a resource that combines serious content with visual appeal. Spread throughout the book are sidebars, photographs, tables, figures, and personal profiles. We've tried to make it easy to read and easy to find the exact information you are looking for. Yet we've retained the solid content and the understanding tone that readers connected with in the first edition.

The book is divided into seven chapters that move more or less chronologically through history and through a woman's life. After an opening section called "Meet the Melpomene Institute," where you find out more about us, the book's first chapter concerns how our culture's understanding of women and physical activity has changed over the years. Active young women today may be surprised to learn how much they owe their female ancestors who paved the way for the revolution that occurred in the 1970s. But we still have a ways to go: Many misconceptions about the female body and physical activity remain intact today.

Chapter 2 deals with body image: how our images of our bodies develop and sometimes become distorted. Discussed here are ways to become comfortable with your own body, individual differences in body composition and metabolism, and considerations regarding dieting and eating habits.

In chapter 3, following a discussion of the benefits of physical activity, we suggest the best ways to choose and start an exercise program, how to keep motivated to continue physical activity, and ways to prevent injury. Information and guidelines are offered for a range of activities, from walking to weight lifting. We inform you of each activity's benefits and tell you how to both start the activity and continue it throughout a long and healthy life.

Chapters 4 and 5 deal with menstruation and pregnancy, two areas where myths about physical activity may cause concern and confusion. Chapter 4 discusses questions active women may have concerning menstruation, while chapter 5 clears up some misconceptions about the active pregnant woman. Both these topics are discussed in light of current research, and practical recommendations are offered.

Chapter 6 focuses on the fitness of your child or children, discussing the benefits of physical activity for children, the factors that determine how active a child will be, and the ways you can encourage the kids in your life to be physically active.

The final chapter in the book is on the natural process of aging. We weigh the factors important to older women who wish to continue exercising and recommend ways to remain healthy and active. We also discuss conditions related to aging, including menopause and osteoporosis, and the benefits physical activity can provide.

We hope that *The Bodywise Woman,* written by women for women, helps you become comfortable with who you are and how you treat yourself.

Meet the Melpomene Institute

When you think of an institute, do you imagine a stately brick manor with white columns and manicured lawns? Or a high-tech laboratory filled with serious people in white coats? Either way, you'd probably be surprised to find our comfortable, sun-filled offices located in St. Paul, Minnesota. Come upstairs and we'll introduce you to the real Melpomene Institute.

We are a network of researchers, educators, and supporters who are dedicated to studying the impact of physical activity on women and girls. We are based in Minnesota, but our 1,900 members hail from every state in the U.S. as well as from Canada and several other countries. Incorporated as a nonprofit agency in 1982, we're proud to have become the nation's leading source of research information on the relationship between women's health and physical activity. Our eight part-time staff members and cadre of interns and trained volunteers conduct research on topics such as osteoporosis, body image, menstrual function, girls and self-esteem, and exercise and pregnancy. We also publish a journal and newsletter, organize educational seminars, maintain a resource library of 4,000 articles, produce videos and informational packets, and give speeches across the country.

Writing *The Bodywise Woman* brought us full circle. The first edition, published in 1990, sold 20,000 copies. The book was created for the same reason we started Melpomene: We wanted to provide up-to-date, unbiased information that would help women make informed choices about their own health and lifestyles. In 1982 we could only dream about the day when there might be enough information about women and exercise to fill a book. There was plenty known about the impact of exercise on the male body, and a few studies looked at elite women athletes on college teams, but for the most part, the average woman who stepped out of her house every morning to run or bike or walk was operating in the dark. If she had questions about why her period had stopped, or whether she could still train for a marathon now that she was pregnant, she had only one place to go—her doctor. Because of the shortage of relevant research, doctors often took a cautious approach: Stop exercising, they suggested, and whatever problems you are experiencing should go away.

For many women who were just starting to feel the freedom, power, and sense of well-being that physical activity provided, this was not an acceptable answer. Judy Mahle Lutter was one of those women. It was 1973, and Judy, a 33-year-old mother of three, was in desperate need of some quiet time. One day when her husband, Hap, a marathon runner, came trotting in from his daily run, Judy met him at the door. "It's my turn," she told him, and before he could react, she was out the door to try running around the block. Until that point, Hap had been the only athlete in the house. Judy had been a chubby kid with the nickname of "Tubs" and had shied away from anything athletic. Slowly but surely, she advanced from barely being able to make it around the block to running her first 26.2-mile marathon 2 years later. By 1978, the year she recorded her personal best of 2:56 at the Boston Marathon, Judy was known around town as the resident expert on women and running.

She began getting calls from women who assumed she would know about everything from nutrition to sports bras to whether or not women runners could get pregnant. Judy, in fact, could not answer their questions with any authority and, for that matter, couldn't locate experts or research that would provide the answers. One of the questions that kept arising concerned irregular menstrual cycles or total loss of periods (amenorrhea). Judy, who holds master's degrees in educational psychology and American studies, decided one way to start getting answers was to do the research herself. She and Pat Weisner, a friend who had coached women athletes for 25 years, devised a brief questionnaire. They polled the local running community. A national sample became possible when two national running publications also printed the questionnaire. To their amazement, 422 women responded.

The most revealing information was due to a printing fluke. Judy and Pat were unable to get all the questions on one side of the page, so they printed the last two on the back of the sheet, with a long blank below. When they invited women to use the area for comments and questions, they had no idea they would receive such lengthy responses. Nearly every woman used the space, and some even stapled extra sheets to the questionnaire. Obviously, physically active women were hungry for some factual information about their own bodies.

As a follow-up, Judy and another friend, medical writer Susan Cushman, devised a second, 12-page questionnaire. It sought information about each woman's running history, menstrual history, contraceptive methods, and physical attributes, and whether she had ever run during a pregnancy. They distributed it at the 1980 Boston Marathon and at the Bonnie Bell all-woman 10K race in the Twin Cities. Data from the 410 respondents suggested that most women runners, contrary to popular opinion, continue to menstruate regularly. Prior to this study, the only research on menstruation had been done on a small group of college athletes who had shown high percentages of amenorrhea (loss of periods). These results made their way into the popular media, leaving the false impression that vigorous exercise always leads to amenorrhea.

The interest generated by the survey convinced Judy and Susan that there was a need for more formal research. In 1982, they incorporated as a nonprofit agency with the mission of linking physical activity to women's health. They named their new institute Melpomene (pronounced Mel-POM-uh-nee), in honor of the Greek woman who defied officials by running the marathon course at the 1896 Olympics after she had been told women could not enter the race. Several accounts exist surrounding her unofficial running of the distance. The most authoritative source states that she participated with the men in a marathon trial. She finished the course in a respectable 4 hours and 30 minutes, becoming the first woman to complete an Olympic marathon.

For the first year, Judy was the only staff person, and she worked part-time on Melpomene while holding down another job. As membership grew and the research projects took on a life of their own, Judy decided to quit her job and give Melpomene her full attention. The timing was right: The running boom was drawing thousands of women who had never before exercised, aerobic dance was beginning to mushroom, and YWCAs and fitness clubs were attracting record numbers of women participants. Each time the Institute's work appeared on television or in the press, the phones would ring off the hook with more questions and more thank-yous from women who were grateful that a group such as Melpomene finally existed.

Melpomene was, and still is, a one-of-a-kind organization. We are unique in at least four ways. First, we focus on research but operate outside of a medical or academic setting. While this independence frees us from certain biases, it also limits our access to traditional granting institutions. Because we are not all physicians or PhDs, we lack the "union card" that would admit us to the more common funding sources. By creatively working with small family foundations and academic experts, we have been able to build an outstanding reputation and attract high-quality sponsors and staff. Our board of directors and advisors includes nationally recognized specialists in sports medicine, gynecology, nutrition, physical education, and psychology. They are active participants, helping to design and direct our multidisciplinary studies. Being outside the usual academic setting has the advantage of allowing us to be more creative and to go directly to our audience to help shape the pertinent research questions.

Our second unique characteristic is that we have access to a population of research subjects (our members) who range from age 7 to 89, and who run the gamut from sideline supporters who are themselves sedentary to gold medal Olympians. Between the two extremes are women who are occasionally active as well as those who try to do something active every day. Some of our members compete in a sport, but most participate purely for fun. The one trait all of our members have in common is a strong belief that physical activity does have a place in a healthy lifestyle. So far, we've conducted three studies directed exclusively at our members: one in 1981-1982, a second in 1984-1985, and a third in 1990. In the first, 197 women filled out detailed questionnaires; in the second, we heard from 420 women. Our most recent study was completed by 672 women. Answers to these three studies provided reams of information about the lifestyles, medical histories, attitudes, and exercise patterns of active and not-so-active women. You'll be reading about some of the results throughout this book.

Our members are not the only people we examine in our research projects. In fact, Melpomene members usually make up less than 10 percent of our sample populations. Most of our research participants learn about our studies by reading about them in newspapers, the Women's Sports Foundation newsletter, and most recently *Self* and *Shape* magazines. Frequently we survey not only physically active participants but also a comparison group of nonactive subjects. In the past three years, national organizations and publications have sought us out, forming partnerships with us to gather and disseminate information of interest to their target audiences.

Over the years other Melpomene studies have looked at populations that have not been examined before, such as seniors, disabled athletes, chemically dependent women, toddlers, teenagers, and large women. These broad, varied sample groups distinguish our studies from those that focus only on women in collegiate or semiprofessional sports programs. Because our samples include women who are older and women who are noncompetitive, our findings apply to a wider range of ages and abilities.

Our studies set us apart in a third way. Rather than isolating one physiological function affected by exercise, our research focuses on the whole woman. We use questionnaires to gather information about eating and sleeping habits, menstrual patterns, medical history, psychological well-being, attitudes toward body image, and patterns of exercise. We also conduct focus groups to help us define the most appropriate questions or further explore findings. On occasion we also use body fat measurements, CT (computerized tomography) scans, dietary analysis, and blood tests; but the strength of our results comes from what we learn about a woman's entire lifestyle.

The ongoing nature of some of our studies is the fourth Melpomene trademark. Women who were enrolled in our osteoporosis study in 1982, for example, have been studied every couple of years since. In 1995 we still had 83 of the original 111 willing to fill out questionnaires. Of the original 111 women, who ranged in age from 46 to 80 at the start of the study, 6 have died, a few have been lost as they moved around the country, and some have lost interest. But the number who continue to provide us with information is encouraging and enlightening. See chapter 7 for more details on our osteoporosis study.

Throughout Melpomene's history we've been interested in taking research information and making it accessible to a large audience. We've made a special point in the past six years, since the first edition of *The Bodywise Woman* was published, to produce educational materials directly related to current research topics. An award-winning video, "Heroes, Growing up Female and Strong," produced by Jane Helmke in conjunction with KARE 11 TV, a Gannett affiliate, used Melpomene research to explore the impact of physical activity on self-esteem for girls. The video has been purchased by hundreds of schools, youth groups, and parents. An accompanying curriculum provides tools for ongoing discussion of the problems girls face and suggests ways they might become more confident and competent.

In addition to producing print publications and videos, we serve as a clearing house and information center. We review scores of journals, newsletters, and abstracts to keep our pulse on current research of interest to physically active women. Our library of more than 4,000 research articles is computerized for easy access. Students, educators, speakers, coaches, and individuals like yourself use our resource center to explore a topic in depth or to answer a specific question. Further, to reach a larger audience we've compiled packets of information on 14 topics. These packets contain the best current articles on a particular subject, updated each year by Melpomene staff. Our readers appreciate the fact that we've mixed research articles with less technical materials and provided summaries and comments to make them user-friendly.

To make our resource center materials available to more members and friends, we've recently created our own bulletin board and gone on-line. It's still too early to measure results, but we expect that the interaction this medium provides will encourage more women to contact us directly.

We've also learned that the media are an important and effective way to get our message to a large audience. In 1994, Judy Mahle Lutter began writing a weekly column in the sports pages of the Sunday St. Paul *Pioneer Press*. In any given year more than 75 articles about our work are published in newspapers, magazines, and newsletters. In excess of 24 million people read about Melpomene. Information about our work appears in the *New York Times*, the *Chicago Tribune, Self, Shape,* and other women's sports and fitness magazines. Melpomene staff also make more than 20 radio and TV appearances yearly.

We've developed an active speakers bureau as well. Our experts make about 40 presentations a year to a variety of professional and lay groups nationwide. As more commercial health-care organizations have developed conferences, we find it is more cost-effective to participate in those endeavors rather than sponsoring our own programs. Instead of conferences, we now hold seminars three or four times a year on topics such as aging, kids, and mothers and daughters.

The role of "seed-planter" has become an increasingly important one for us. Since we ourselves cannot tackle all the research questions or reach all the audiences, we have tried to ask questions and raise issues that other organizations can pursue. When we began, we were the only group that was doing research on health-care concerns of physically active women; today we are pleased to report that new research studies are being undertaken every day. This book is an attempt to compile what's known about these topics, combining both our research and the research of others. Even as this book goes to press, there will be new findings that we won't be able to include. Instead of giving you pat answers, therefore, we've tried to give you the tools to evaluate new information as you receive it. Thus, what you learn here need not become obsolete.

Now that we've told you something about ourselves, we'd like to learn more about you. We've found that while lab tests and statistics can produce certain kinds of knowledge, our most valuable findings still come from the experiences of other women. We invite you to send us your questions and comments as you read this book.

We're thrilled to be able to pass this knowledge on to you. The rewriting process for this second edition caused us to carefully reread and update the changes of the past six years. While some advances have clearly been made, more research is clearly needed. In the first edition we asked readers to write us with questions and comments. Many of those suggestions are included here. We extend that invitation again. We also invite you to keep in touch with our latest developments by becoming a member by writing the Melpomene

Institute at 1010 University Avenue, St. Paul, MN 55104. Or give us a call at 612-642-1951 or send a fax to 612-642-1871. You can also reach us by e-mail at Melpomene@Webspan.com. Better yet, next time you're in the heartland, why not come upstairs and meet our "institute" in person!

—The Staff and Researchers of the
Melpomene Institute for Women's Health Research

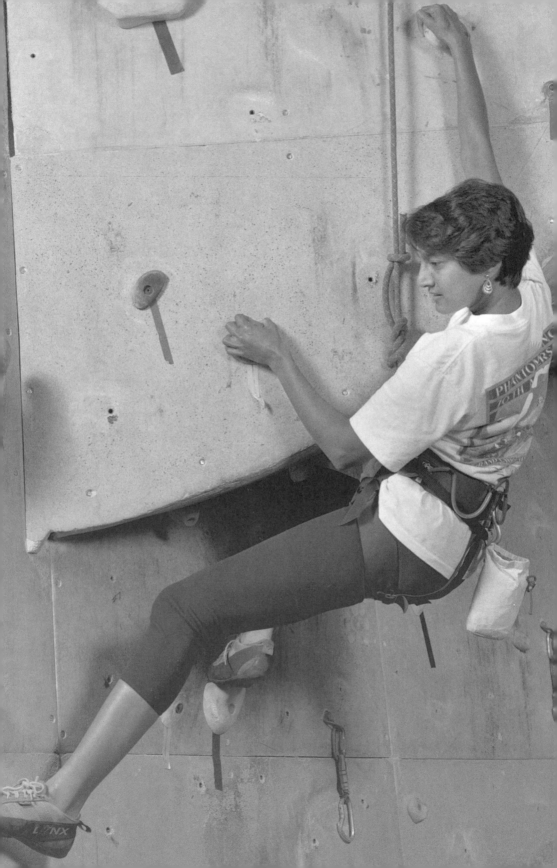

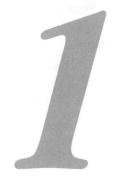

How Far We've Come: A Historical Look at Women and Exercise

Our mothers are amazed. We're winning racquetball tournaments, running marathons, swimming miles before work, and climbing mountains with our bikes. We're exercising in larger numbers than any previous generation of women. Finally our time has come to share in the joys and exhilaration of excelling, achieving, and transforming our self-image through sport. Now that we know how good it feels to be active, we can't help but wonder: What took us so long?

The acceptance of women in sport has not followed a steady, uphill course throughout history. Instead, it has gone through many peaks and valleys—times when female sports figures were popular heroines and times when athletic women were condemned as unfit mothers. Examination of the historical settings illuminates the influence of society in the sport arena, and a pattern begins to emerge. It seems that a shift in society's priorities nearly always comes just before or behind the major movements in women's sports. Women have either been welcomed or barred from sports depending on what society needed or wanted them to be at the time. When a healthy "Rosie the Riveter" was needed during World War II, for instance, strength and physical activity were patriotic. Then, when men returned and wanted women back at home, a rash of articles about the "dangers" of exercise appeared. Acceptance of athletic women seemingly has come and gone depending on what kind of woman society favors at the time.

The media and the medical profession have often worked hand-in-hand to shape opinions and carry out particular agendas. Medical authorities are still called on to either hail the benefits of physical activity or issue grave warnings against sport for women. Historically, misinformation kept women in bed during their periods and made them feel guilty about exercising for fear of what it would do to their reproductive organs. Decades of myths remain to be dispelled. To understand how these myths began, it helps to go back and look at the societal trends that dictated acceptance of or resistance to women in sport.

CORSETS AND CLASSISM—
THE VICTORIAN ERA

The nineteenth century was a period of paradox in terms of women and their bodies. Immigrants from Europe were reaching our eastern shores in droves, while at the western edge of the nation pioneer women were hacking homesteads out of the raw wilderness. For these women, the question of what to do with leisure time was moot: Survival was a full-time pursuit, and women were run ragged with 14-hour-a-day industrial jobs, or with chopping wood, hauling water, growing crops, herding livestock, tending to children, and building homes. Enslaved black women survived and persisted in spite of the intense physical labor demanded of them. For each of these groups, physical strength and endurance was a valued commodity and posed no challenge to a woman's femininity or fertility. On the contrary, the working class woman *depended* on her body for survival.

At the same time, middle-class and upper-class urban women were striving to appear as physically weak and helpless as they could in order to achieve "true womanhood." The "true woman," according to Victorian ideals, was passive, frail, delicate, ethereal, and soft. She was elevated onto a moral pedestal and was the keeper of her husband's last refuge—a calm, peaceful household where he could come home and forget the struggles of the outside world. To maintain her purity, the Victorian woman was urged to stay indoors, safe from the world's evils. Of course, for women who operated machines, worked in the fields, hand-washed clothing, and toiled over kitchen stoves, this ideal was beyond reach. The only women who could actually attain this pedestal (although all were taught to aspire to it) were those of the middle and upper classes.

Because a woman could belong to this leisure class only by attaching herself to a man, it was imperative that the Victorian woman be attractive at all times. She cultivated a white pallor with the fervor that some modern women reserve for tanning, and with the help of corsets, she achieved the illusion of having a delicate, tiny waist. No matter what size she was originally, a woman could use the wire or whalebone garment to reduce her waist by 2 to 8 inches. Some women even had ribs removed so they could cinch themselves tighter. This abdominal equivalent of Chinese foot binding exerted an average of 21 pounds of pressure on internal organs, restricting circulation and displacing the liver, spleen, intestines, and bladder. If you also consider that the well-dressed woman sported up to 37 pounds of street clothing in the winter (19 pounds of which was suspended from her waist), you can begin to understand why she fainted so often!

Ironically, the dress of the day hindered one of the primary "functions" of the Victorian lady—motherhood. Many miscarriages were caused by tightly laced corsets, and in extreme cases, a woman's uterus could actually collapse and be forced through her vagina. Because of the prevailing societal beliefs, a reproductive failure such as this was the worst thing that could happen to a woman.

A Woman Is Her Uterus

A large part of the Victorian woman's mystery was what lay beneath the yards of petticoats; her ability to give birth was what made her a creature composed of "finer clay" than her husband. The reproductive organs were therefore central to a woman's entire being, and the medical community believed that all sicknesses, from headaches to heart conditions to insanity, could be traced to her uterus or her ovaries. In 1849, Dr. Frederick Hollick wrote in his book *The Diseases of Women, Their Cause and Cure Familiarly Explained*:

> The uterus, it must be remembered, is the *controlling* organ in the female body, being the most excitable of all, and so is ultimately connected, by the ramifications of its numerous nerves, with every other part. (Ehrenreich and English, 1978)

Dr. M.E. Dirix concurred in 1869, writing in *Woman's Complete Guide to Health*:

> Thus women are treated for diseases of the stomach, liver, kidneys, heart, lungs, etc.; yet, in most instances, these diseases will be found on due investigation, to be, in reality, no diseases at all, but merely the sympathetic reactions or the symptoms of one disease, namely, a disease of the womb. (ibid., 122)

Perhaps because they knew so little about healthy reproductive functioning, the doctors of that time assumed that the female system was "inherently pathological," and that a woman's natural state was to be sick (ibid., 110). Menstruation, for instance, was seen as a serious threat throughout life. Dr. Engelmann, the president of the American Gynecological Society, was quoted as saying in 1900:

> Many a young life is battered and forever crippled on the breakers of puberty; if it crosses these unharmed and is not dashed to pieces on the rock of childbirth, it may still ground on the ever-recurring shallows of menstruation, and lastly upon the final bar of the menopause ere protection is found on the unruffled waters of the harbor beyond reach of sexual storms (ibid., 110).

According to the "experts," only a man of medicine could help a woman navigate through the dangerous waters of her life. Thus, the household doctor was an indispensable figure in upper-class families and he was paid handsomely to "manage" the woman's many illnesses. Women were taught to trust their doctor's every word. When it came to recreational activities, the doctor's orders were to get outside, enjoy the fresh air, socialize with others of one's class, but avoid breaking into an indelicate sweat. Genteel sports of archery, croquet, bowling, tennis, and golf were the primary activities and were usually associated with the opportunity to have respectable social encounters. Swimming was also purported to be therapeutic, but only if performed in concordance with Victorian mores of modesty and propriety.

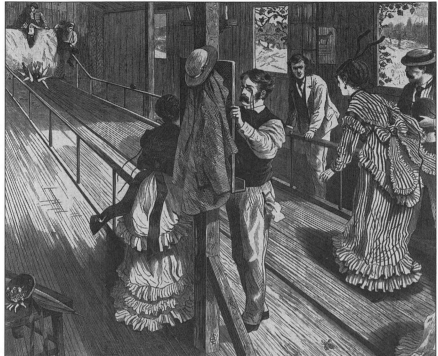

© Courtesy Sally Fox

This drawing, from an 1869 edition of *Harpers*, shows a public bowling match in New England. Women bowlers regularly competed against men as well as against other women.

Because the Victorians believed that the human body was indecent, both men's and women's fashions were designed to keep the maximum amount of skin covered. Of course, this idea made swimming on a public beach difficult. After struggling with how to allow women to swim and yet not bare their skin, society came up with a compromise that was more like bathing than what we think of as swimming. A woman would enter a wooden box on the beach and change into a full-length dress that was somewhat more comfortable, but certainly not more revealing, than her usual wardrobe. The wooden box would then be rolled into the water, where, beyond the eyes of the public, she could emerge and dunk herself. The impracticality of this arrangement was obvious to one male swimming instructor who wrote in 1903:

> Just to satisfy myself on this point of costume, I once wore a close approximation of the usual suit for women. Not until then did I rightly understand what a serious matter a few feet of superfluous cloth might become in water. The suit was amply large, yet pounds

of apparently dead weight seemed to be pulling me in every direction. In that gear a swim of one hundred yards was as serious a task as a mile in my own suit. After that experience, I no longer wondered why so few women really swim well, but rather that they are able to swim at all. (Howell 1982, 180)

Although more doctors were beginning to counsel women to exercise, they all agreed that activity had to cease during the "sexual storms" of a woman's menstrual period. In 1871, Dr. W.C. Taylor gave a typical warning in his book *A Physician's Counsels to Woman in Health and Disease:*

> We cannot too emphatically urge the importance of regarding these monthly returns as periods of ill health, as days when the ordinary occupations are to be suspended or modified . . . Long walks, dancing, shopping, riding and parties should be avoided at this time of month invariably and under all circumstances . . ." (Ehrenreich and English 1978, 111)

When it came to pregnancy, the warnings were particularly loud. A woman was considered "indisposed" for the entire 9 months before the birth of her child, and after the delivery she was advised to "recuperate" by lying in bed for many more months. These prescriptions did not seem to apply to working-class women, however. Employers gave no time off for pregnancy or recovery from childbirth, much less for painful menstrual periods. No matter how sick she was, a woman risked losing her job if she missed one day of work. Slave women, of course, did not have jobs to lose; instead, they could be beaten or otherwise severely punished for missing work. The old belief that the underclasses were somehow biologically different came in handy. As Barbara Ehrenreich and Deidre English note in their book *For Her Own Good:*

> *Someone* had to be well enough to do the work, though, and working-class women, Dr. Warner (a popular medical authority writing in 1874) noted with relief, were *not* invalids: "The African Negress, who toils beside her husband in the fields of the south, and Bridget, who washes, and scrubs and toils in our homes at the north, enjoy for the most part good health, with comparative immunity from uterine disease." (ibid., 114)

"Brain Fever Threatens Womanhood"

The absurdity of these contradictions was becoming obvious to many women who began to see that they restricted not only their physical activity, but also their freedom. The suffrage movement was gaining momentum, and more and more middle-class women were seeking ways to improve themselves. They enrolled in women's colleges such as Smith (opened in 1872), Wellesley (1875), Bryn Mawr (1885), and Mills (1885) and even fought to enter the all-male bastions such as Cornell and Harvard.

Higher education for women was viewed as a great experiment. Many believed that the stresses of study and life away from doctor's supervision would prove too much for the frail female composition. As Dr. Edward H. Clarke said in his widely read tract called "Sex in Education, or a Fair Chance for the Girls," the female system is not able to do two things well at once. He subscribed to a popular belief that the body was like a miniature economy and that various parts of the body were competing for a limited pool of resources. When a woman studied, he explained, blood would be diverted to her brain, robbing essential organs of a precious life force. The organ that was in direct competition with the brain, of course, was the uterus. Clarke's book, which was so popular it had to be reprinted 17 times, warned that higher education would cause a woman's uterus to atrophy.

To prevent this catastrophe, the founders of women's colleges instituted a program of physical culture that would strengthen the women to help them endure the stresses of college life. Of course, this physical culture had to be of a moderate nature, because too much physical excitement could certainly produce a nervous condition, hysteria, or, even worse, a disruption of menstrual periods. The focus of the activities was on fresh air, cooperation, hygiene, and posture. Walking was most strongly encouraged as training for wifely duties such as washing, cleaning, and gardening. Other college sports included golf, tennis, croquet, archery, gymnastics, rowing, and swimming.

Women physical educators were hired to guide these activities and ensure that women did not overexert themselves or risk possible disfigurement through too much bodily contact. Endurance sports such as track and field were discouraged because they would produce more "physical straining than physical training," a phrase coined by Mabel Lee, a typical physical educator of this period. Likewise, basketball was modified to minimize the possible danger of contact. The court was divided into thirds, and players (six to a team) had to stay in their third. The number of dribbles was limited, and the rules penalized even accidental brushes.

Guardians of Femininity—Physical Educators and the Anticompetition Movement

Safeguarding the health of their students was only one aspect of the physical educators' job. They believed that their higher calling was to

Barbara Andersen: Going Strong

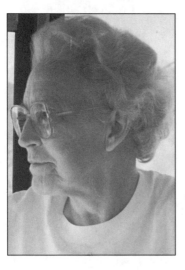

"Although I haven't played softball for forty years, my body still knows the feel of the sharp grounder hitting my glove at third base, the automatic shifting of my feet, the fluid movement of whipping the ball to first base and the satisfying 'pop' of the ball in the first baseman's glove."

At 71, **Barbara Andersen,** a college professor who teaches writing, has many memories to share. "As a child I never heard, 'girls don't do this, girls don't do that'. I think that's one reason I've always been physically active: I was never programmed not to be." Barbara learned to play softball in a vacant lot. Her instructors were the young adult men of the neighborhood. "They made no distinction between the younger boys and girls. At first you stood on the sidelines and watched and learned. Then you'd get a chance to run for a batter. If you were lucky, they'd teach you to bat. Finally, girl or boy, if you had paid your dues, you became a ball player."

As a teenager, Barbara played softball in one of the many city leagues for young women that provided girls with the same opportunities to play as the boys had in their leagues. At her high school, however, Barbara noticed differences in the way male and female athletes were treated. "Girls could play basketball but couldn't play full court. When you got to the center line, you threw the ball to a teammate on the other side. Female organs, you know. The boys played the other schools and got a lot of press; the girls were restricted to intramurals." Unfortunately, things only got worse: In college, Barbara had almost no opportunity for sports except for pickup games of softball and basketball.

Barbara remained active, biking and walking for exercise until she was 50. Then she joined a women's health club. "I started running at age 55 and racing at 60. I had no idea when I started that there were other women my age running."

In the last few years, Barbara has taken up camping, canoeing, and weight training. "I don't see any reason for not trying new things just because you're older. It's true I can't actually play softball anymore, but," she grins, "I'll always be a softball player in my heart."

safeguard the feminine, moral nature of their students and to keep them from falling prey to the "treacheries of competition" that "sullied" men's sports. They believed that competition bred aggressiveness and encouraged individual excellence, both of which were out of step with woman's "inborn sense of modesty and innocence." Once an athlete was singled out as a star, they argued, she would be vulnerable to commercial exploitation: People might offer her scholarships or pay to see her perform. Publicity associated with success would also violate the ideal that a woman should be unobtrusive. As one physical educator of the time noted, "The development of aggressive characteristics . . . added nothing to charm and usefulness, and were not in harmony with the best traditions of the sex." The aesthetic appeal of sports was important: We should worry about looking pretty rather than winning.

By de-emphasizing individual excellence, the physical educators truly believed they were performing a service and providing the greatest good for the greatest number. They also felt that women, who were believed to be morally superior to men, must uphold the feminine ideal. Unfortunately, these educators' loyalty to an antiquated, and in many ways harmful, ideal blinded them to the realities of the quickly changing world. As unbelievable as it seems, many physical educators fought strongly to exclude women from the Olympics from 1896 to 1932. But, thanks to events occurring in the larger world outside of college campuses, they found themselves fighting a rising tide of support for women in sports.

SUFFRAGETTES AND BICYCLES

Despite the objections of some social commentators and medical authorities, sports were about to break out of the country clubs and college campuses and become available to many more women. A number of factors contributed to the softening of society's taboos against women's sports. The suffrage movement was gaining momentum, more women were entering the world of work, and a few glamorous sportswomen were starting to achieve fame. Slowly but surely, the spell of the Victorian ideal was starting to lose its power.

The invention of the bicycle around the year 1870 proved to be a crucial factor. Suddenly, an acceptable form of physical activity was available to women. The relaxation of fashion standards was perhaps one of the most revolutionary effects of the bicycle's arrival. Skirts too were suddenly no longer practical. Bloomers, which had been invented and considered outrageous 50 years before, finally became

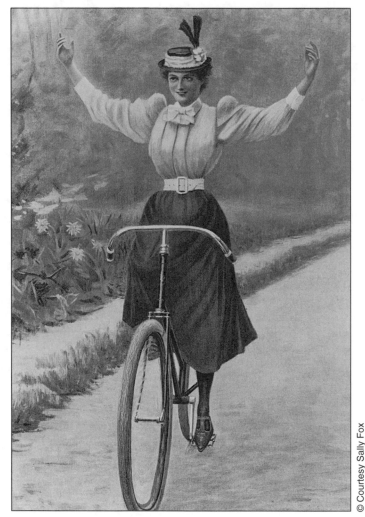

© Courtesy Sally Fox

In the late 1800s women apparently were not discouraged from riding bicycles—even though this often meant trading their skirts for bloomers.

acceptable garb not only on the bike but also in many public places. A craze swept the country, and by 1896 an estimated four million riders were using their bikes for transportation as well as for exercise.

As always, a few dissenting voices tried to stem the tide of this new fad. Some insisted that bicycle riding would induce sexual sensations, driving virtuous women to prostitution. Others sang the old song about bike seats being harmful to women's reproductive organs. This time, women didn't listen; they abandoned their petticoats, took to their bikes, and continued to have healthy babies.

THE EMERGENCE OF TEAM AND INDIVIDUAL SPORTS

Games such as basketball became popular, but, as noted earlier, the rules were changed to make distances shorter and activity less strenuous in order to protect the femininity of women. In 1912, Dr. Dudley Allen Sargent was quoted as saying it was fine for women to be athletes, but performing "men's athletics" made women more masculine. Albert Spalding, whose name has become synonymous with sporting equipment, was also in favor of women competing in sports, as long as they didn't invade some sacred male domains. The national pastime, for instance, was to be off-limits to women. In 1911, he said:

> Neither our wives, our daughters, nor our sweethearts may play Base Ball on the field. They may play Cricket, but seldom do; they may play Lawn Tennis and win championships; they may play Basket Ball, and achieve laurels; they may play Golf, and receive trophies; but Base Ball is too strenuous for womankind, except as she may take part in the grandstand. (Howell 1982, 186)

World War I became the catalyst for new attitudes. Women were encouraged to work in factories to support the war effort. The medical community suggested exercise as an antidote to the long hours and poor working conditions in most factories, so these women were also introduced to recreation and sports teams organized by their employers. While the best facilities and the greatest number of teams were for men, some companies had very active women's programs. For the first time, the nation was introduced to athletes from the working class. Mildred "Babe" Didrickson, who went on to set world records in the 1932 Olympics and achieve excellence and fame in many sports, came out of this tradition.

Many of the gains achieved by women during World War I persisted into the 1920s. Standards were relaxed, and women enjoyed a new autonomy. Winning the right to vote triggered a social release and made women feel as if their lives were changing. The number of women in the labor force was 26 percent higher than at any previous time in American history. Moreover, many women were living away from home for the first time in order to be close to work. This large, new pool of women had the money and leisure time to engage in a whole host of new sports: volleyball, softball, field hockey, bowling, lacrosse, polo, fencing, swimming, skating, diving, and even sailboat racing and flying. Participants were no longer just from the upper classes, although there was some division by class depending on how expensive activities were. Industrial teams continued to be popular, and the opportunities multiplied when municipal recreation departments and agencies such as the YWCA opened for women.

The period from 1920 to the beginning of World War II brought huge gains for women in sport. It was during this time that many sportswomen began to be nationally applauded for their prowess. Glenna Collett, for instance, the first woman to break 80 in a round of golf, won her first of six amateur championships in 1922 at the age of 19. In 1926, Gertrude Ederle became the first woman to swim across the English Channel, breaking the male world record by 2 hours. Helen Wills, known as "Little Miss Poker Face," dominated the tennis scene for most of the 1920s and into the 1930s. She won seven U.S. singles titles at Forest Hills, eight Wimbledon titles, and a gold medal at the 1928 Paris Olympics.

PLAY DAYS WIN OUT OVER COMPETITION

Meanwhile, as women's sports were quickly gaining in popularity in the world at large, female physical educators were still trying to keep women from competitive activity. They felt more strongly than ever that women should not follow the men's pattern of intercollegiate competition. Commercialization, they feared, was like a "malignant growth which would eat at the soul of sports." In 1923, the newly formed Woman's Division of the National Amateur Athletic Federation passed a platform that shrunk what few opportunities there were for women to compete against their counterparts at other colleges. The physical educators cited men coaches, unchaperoned travel arrangements, questionable uniforms, and the inappropriate use of women in sport advertising as the reasons for curtailing intercollegiate competition.

In its place, schools developed play days. The idea of a play day was to bring together women from a number of schools for a day of sports and recreational activities. The day included relays where everyone participated as well as games such as net ball, hockey, swimming, and basketball where some participated while others cheered. Individual schools would not compete against each other, but rather, each team would be composed of women from various schools. This way, supposedly, they would get to know one another but avoid the competitive feelings that an established team would be able to form. Frequent breaks for juice and cookies prevented the players from overexerting themselves and gave them time to socialize. According to the University of California Women's Athletic Association, the play days allowed women to "carry away a feeling of group loyalty and unmarred fellow-ship," which was more important than excelling as an individual.

Not everyone was enamored with the system, however. Eleanor Metheny, a physical educator who had grown up during the era of play days, reflected on the stigma attached to the concept of winning:

> We had fun at those play days, and we enjoyed the tea and the sociability—but the better players among us felt frustrated by the lack of meaningful team play . . . These play days did little to satisfy our desire for all-out competition with worthy and honored opponents. (Howell 1982, 255)

Both the Committee of Women's Athletics and the Women's Division of the National Amateur Athletic Federation continued to support such events and to oppose programs such as the Olympic games, which they considered improper. They approved of athletics "motivated by joy and love of play, not for the purpose of making a record or beating an opponent." Although both of these groups resisted efforts to send women to the Olympics in 1928, and again in 1932, they were unsuccessful. By that time, women had already begun to make inroads into sporting history.

THE DEPRESSION BURSTS THE BUBBLE

The women's sports movement suffered a setback when the Depression hit in the thirties. Suddenly, it was seen as unpatriotic to take a man's place in a job. Fewer women worked, went to college, or could afford to live away from home. With their freedom compromised, and the nation becoming somewhat more conservative, scientific evidence appeared to help escort women back to their traditional roles as home-maker and mother. In 1936, an article appearing in the prestigious *Scientific American* warned that "feminine muscular development interferes with motherhood."

Questions about athletes' femininity were also raised. People could not understand women such as Mildred "Babe" Didrickson, whose physical capabilities appeared to match those of a man. The gossip about Didrickson was vicious, and even lacy clothes and a marriage did little to quell the rumors. In 1936, Lewis Terman wrote a book entitled *Sex and Personality*, in which he presented a scale that would presumably enable clinicians to determine how feminine or masculine their clients were. Curiously, he chose a scoring system that assigned negative numbers to feminine traits and positive numbers to masculine traits. Therefore, the average woman might have a score in the negative 50s, whereas an average male might score in the plus 50s. Terman found that "highly intelligent, athletic women" had scores closer to the male range than any other group of women, and scored as more "masculine" than male artists. The information fed right into the hands of those who wanted to believe that sportswomen were unnatural and/ or that sports participation would make a woman more masculine.

The medical misinformation and the psychological scare tactics seemed to be working. Fewer women were joining sports leagues, and the new gymnasiums built through federal post-Depression programs were rarely filled with women.

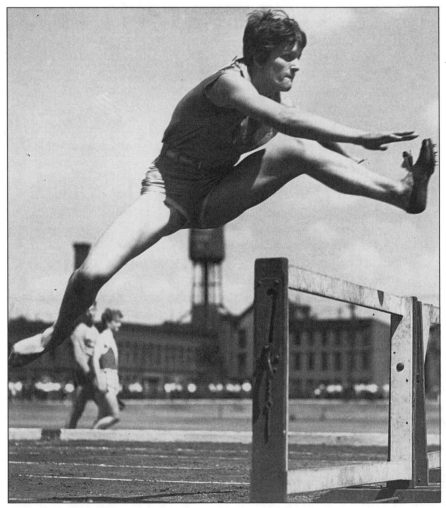

Mildred "Babe" Didrickson in 1931.

EXERCISE BECOMES PATRIOTIC AGAIN— THE WORLD WAR II ERA

This time-out didn't last long. America's entry into the Second World War once again changed society's attitude toward women. With millions of men in Europe, factories were desperate for workers to meet the escalating demands for supplies. Suddenly, it became not only acceptable for women to work but downright patriotic.

Four million women entered the labor force between 1940 and 1942, and they shattered assumptions about what women could do mentally

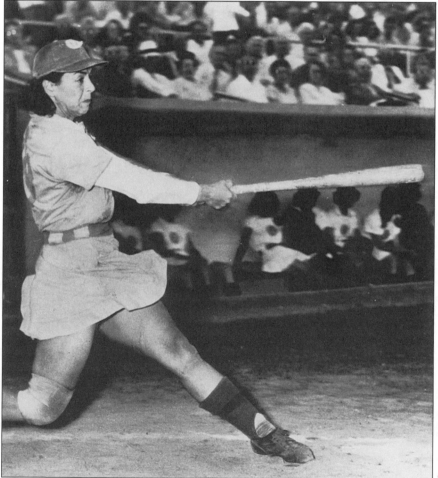

Courtesy of National Baseball Library & Archive, Cooperstown, NY

The first women's baseball league flourished in the 1940s—but when the war ended and the men came home, the league folded.

and physically. Women were drafting, driving trucks, riveting steel, and building battleships. Even in the military, wartime urgency was pushing women through doors that had never been open before. Women filled many noncombative positions in Europe, again to free males for fighting. For the first time, images of strong, able-bodied women were displayed as positive examples. It was quite a departure from the fixation on weak, passive, obedient housewives of a generation before!

One of the unique results of men's absence in this country was the formation of an all-women's professional baseball league. Phillip Wrigley, owner of the Chicago Cubs, decided to see if women athletes could fill a stadium and thus fill the vacuum left by the break in men's pro ball. His gamble paid off, and the league was tremendously popular. The players were chosen for a combination of their baseball skill and feminine characteristics. The hems of their uniforms could be no more than 6 inches above the knee, which, when you think about it, was quite a measure of progress from the days when field hockey dresses could be only 6 inches from the ground! The league managed to last for 12 years, when it finally lost out to the return of the men's game, TV, and strong social pressure for women to once again return to home and hearth.

CHANGES FOLLOWING WORLD WAR II

Shortly after World War II, the Amateur Athletic Union conducted a study of the effects of athletic competition on girls and women. Using a single quote from a female doctor as evidence, the organization concluded that competition during a woman's period might have a harmful effect on a woman's capacity for "being a normal mother." Even in the 1950s, the play day was still the most popular form of competition on most college campuses. The opportunities for sporting challenges that women had enjoyed during the war were effectively placed on the back burner until later in the century. For the time being, "Father Knows Best" was on TV, and Dr. Spock was telling mothers how to be mothers.

THE DRIVE FOR EQUALITY— THE MODERN ERA

It wasn't until the 1960s and 1970s that women once again began to fight for their right to participate equally in sports opportunities, as both amateurs and professionals. They watched from the sidelines as the world of men's athletics mushroomed into the multibillion-dollar industry that it is today. The increased emphasis on sport careers affected every level of competition, enabling thousands of men to compete in high-stakes college athletics and then go on to make their living as professional athletes.

When women first began banging at the door to this "sportsworld," they encountered plenty of opposition. At schools where they succeeded in obtaining official support for teams, their budgets were typically anemic compared with those of men's teams. When Vassar went co-ed in 1969, for instance, the school created a budget for men's athletics that was twice the size of the women's, in spite of the fact that enrollment was still two-thirds women!

Without a strong history of women's achievements in the 1920s and 1930s, women once again had to prove that they were capable in athletics. Unfortunately, their opportunities to train and excel were limited. Women were still excluded from many sports in the Olympics, including pole vaulting, weight lifting, high hurdles, and all forms of team games except volleyball. In her 1965 book *Connotations of Movement in Sport and Dance*, Eleanor Metheny theorized that women were being excluded because society didn't want women competing in sports with the potential for body contact and the need to physically subdue an opponent. Once again, men were busy protecting women's reproductive organs and femininity!

Thankfully, the blossoming women's rights and civil rights movements were giving people the courage to ignore societal rules while they worked to change them. In the 1960s talented athletes such as Willye White and Wilma Rudolph proved that women belonged in the Olympics. They also became powerful role models for black girls. Lisa Lissimore, associate director of the Minnesota State High School League, first learned about Wilma when she was in fifth grade.

> "She made me proud to be an African-American. I realized that she was the type of human being I aspire to be most like. Not because she was the first American woman to win three gold Olympic medals, but because of her majestic dignity. To me, Wilma symbolized the inspiration, the courage, and the endurance to hurdle life's obstacles."

In 1967 Kathrine Switzer entered the Boston Marathon as K. Switzer. Women were not allowed to run in the event, and when officials discovered "K" running the race, they tried to bodily remove her. She slipped past them, however, and ran right into the history books. Regardless of Kathrine's successful finish, amateur athletic organizations still did not believe women were capable of running distance events. It was not until 1972 that women were "allowed" to compete in marathons.

Many believe the greatest emancipating event for sporting women came on September 20, 1973. Tennis player Billie Jean King had agreed to duel it out with one of the greatest self-proclaimed male chauvinists of all time, Bobby Riggs. Riggs, himself a tennis player of note, was sure he would win. The contest was quickly billed as a battle of the sexes. Billie Jean dominated the play, winning the three-out-of-five-set match in three straight. Billie Jean was ranked number one in the world five times and number one in the U.S. seven times. She also won 20 Wimbledon championships. Her professional tennis career set the stage for her continued efforts as an outspoken advocate for women's sports. It is largely because of Billie Jean's efforts that women are today

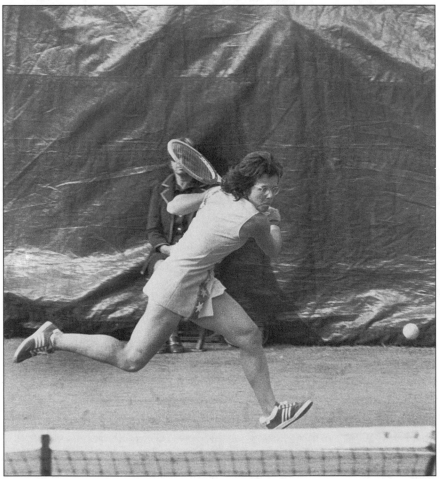

© UPI/Corbis-Bettman

September 20, 1973—Billie Jean King beats Bobby Riggs in three straight sets.

earning lucrative purses in well-publicized tennis events. She continues to be a forceful advocate of women's participation in sports at all levels of play.

TITLE IX: A LANDMARK DECISION

While individual women were breaking barriers, legal clout was necessary to realize many of the gains we currently enjoy. The impetus for change came in 1972 with the enactment of Title IX . This legislation prohibited discrimination on the basis of sex in educational programs that receive federal funds (thus including most of the academic institutions in the country). Athletic programs, which were known for glaring inequities, received new scrutiny. When Title IX took effect for secondary and postsecondary schools in 1978, schools could no longer deny women the right to facilities, budgets, coaches, and uniforms. It did not say that institutions had to match men's and women's programs dollar for dollar, however, nor was it intended to benefit just women. Under Title IX, men could also lobby to form teams that hadn't often existed in a school, such as men's field hockey or volleyball.

Title IX was a monumental landmark that did not go unchallenged. Granted, in the first years after its enactment, schools began increasing opportunities for women, adding to the number of sports offered and allocating more resources to sports for women. The discrepancies were too vast to change quickly, but there was movement toward more equity. However, women's sports suffered a setback in 1984 when the Supreme Court ruled in *Grove City College vs. Bell* that Title IX applied only to specific programs that received federal funding, not entire institutions—effectively ruling that schools did not have to comply with Title IX. As a result, many institutions dropped the reforms they had adopted, and investigations of compliance with Title IX stalled.

Congress turned the situation around, though, when it overrode a presidential veto to pass the Civil Rights Restoration Act in 1988. Then, in 1992 the Supreme Court handed down a ruling that increased Title IX's clout even more. Previously, a finding of noncompliance with Title IX resulted only in an order for the school to comply, by adding a women's team for a sport, increasing resources for recruitment, or otherwise. In the 1992 ruling the Court said that monetary damages may be sought and awarded in Title IX lawsuits. Schools thus have an even larger incentive to ensure compliance, and students who experience discrimination are more likely to pursue their cases, since they can now pay lawyers to represent them.

As the impact of Title IX continues to be felt, schools are increasing their efforts to make athletic opportunities for men and women more equal. The Big Ten, for instance, has mandated that 40 percent of the athletes at all of its member schools be women by June 30, 1997, and the National Collegiate Athletic Association (NCAA) has created a Gender Equity Task Force which has the mission of developing proposals and recommendations to help schools achieve equal opportunity for women in intercollegiate athletics. Understand that gender equity does not mean the same sports for both genders, nor does it mean exactly equal numbers of athletes or identical budgets. It does mean that the available sports and competition levels should accommodate the interests and ability levels of both women and men, and that equipment, facilities, coaching, and other resources are important factors in providing opportunities for students to participate in athletics.

As schools move to make their programs more equitable, they come up against the reality of finite resources. Adding programs for women—programs that were previously nonexistent—means that sometimes less funding is available for other programs. Tempers flare as male coaches complain about the unfairness of seeing their programs squeezed out. Supporters of women's athletic programs hate to see changes that eliminate male sports, but they aren't backing down from claiming their fair share. Christine Grant, women's athletic director at the University of Iowa, said, "It's unfortunate for the young men who get cut, but it's even more unfortunate for the millions of young women who have missed out for 100 years." Supporters of gender equity also point out the little attention that non-revenue sports and walk-ons got until enforcement became an issue.

Another controversial effect of Title IX has been the sharp decline in the number of women coaches and athletic directors in college athletics. One cause of this is the consolidation of men's and women's athletics programs, a step that many schools, ironically, have taken in their move toward compliance with Title IX. Instead of having a women's and a men's athletic director, there is an athletic director and an assistant director. In the vast majority of cases the athletic director is male.

The debate continues over what constitutes compliance with Title IX and how it should be achieved, but the extent of the backlash against equity between the sexes in sports tells us that although it may sometimes feel as if we are in another Golden Age, we may be only at a peak in the ever-changing story of women and sports in America. The value of history is to remind us to take none of our freedoms for granted.

Decline of Women Coaches Since Title IX

Players

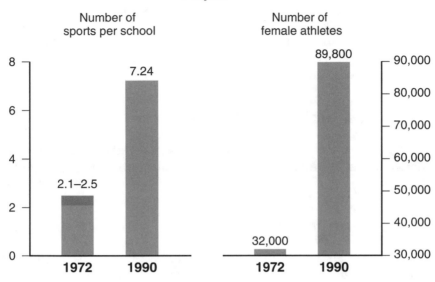

Number of
sports per school

Number of
female athletes

Coaches

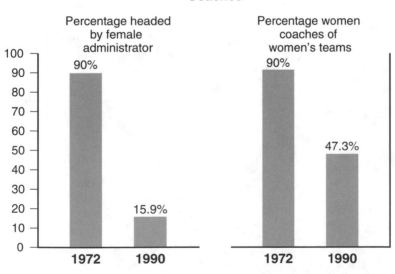

Percentage headed
by female
administrator

Percentage women
coaches of
women's teams

WHERE ARE WE NOW?

In the last 20 years, the medical profession has decided that physical activity is a necessary component of healthy lifestyles for both sexes. More research has been done on exercise in the past decade than in all previous decades combined, and much of it has shown that women are capable of exercise and benefit from it in the same ways that men do.

New Research/New Acceptance

New newspaper columns and magazines devoted to a variety of participatory sports and to health in general have disseminated many of these findings to the general public.

Misleading Information

Because research has traditionally focused on male subjects, much of what is being written about women today is brand new information. Even as you read this book you'll be seeing new studies and information related to women and physical activity. We suggest that you read

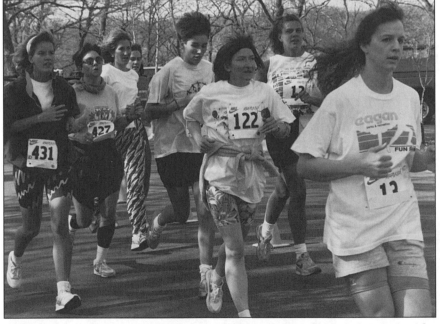

© Melpomene Journal/Mary Lee Slettehaugh

Today almost everyone accepts the idea that the female body is as suited for physical activity as the male body.

the popular press coverage carefully. You may not be getting the complete or accurate story. Hungry for information, reporters sometimes run with stories prematurely, giving impressions that are often misleading and cause women to unnecessarily restrict their physical activity.

An example is the reaction to "Safety Guidelines for Women Who Exercise" released by the American College of Obstetricians and Gynecologists (ACOG) in the spring of 1985. The guidelines recommended 15 to 60 minutes of aerobic activity, 3 to 5 days per week, at 60 percent to 90 percent of aerobic capacity for pregnant women. Quite correctly, the guidelines cautioned women to build up to vigorous activity gradually: "A given level of intensity, duration, and frequency may be safe for a well-conditioned woman but hazardous for one who is deconditioned."

These guidelines were talking about minimum fitness levels for pregnant women who were just starting an exercise program, and were not directed to elite athletes or even recreational athletes. And yet some reporters missed these subtleties. Headlines such as "Docs Tell Women: Go Easy on Exercise" and "Curbs Urged on Exercise for Women" implied that women who were exercising more than three times a week were doing too much. To try to clarify the issue Melpomene and the Women's Sport Foundation coauthored a press release which stated: "There is no reason for pregnant women to limit their exercise to this small quantity. Recreational athletes may choose to exercise for much greater amounts and competitive athletes will need to."

Unfortunately, the ACOG guidelines became the "gold standard" for most physicians and midwives. They worried about medical-legal implications if they recommended higher levels of exercise during pregnancy. While some physicians spoke privately about the unnecessary restrictions imposed by the guidelines, few were willing to encourage higher levels of activity professionally. In 1994 ACOG issued new guidelines which state: "There are no data in humans to indicate that pregnant women should limit exercise intensity or lower target heart rates because of potential adverse effects."

Another example of poor and sometimes sensational reporting accompanied the ideas presented by a panel of experts of the American College of Sports Medicine (ACSM) which met in June 1992. The 2-day workshop addressed disordered eating, menstrual dysfunction, and osteoporosis. The panel identified this constellation of disorders as the Female Athlete Triad. The purpose of the meeting and importance of dealing with the issue were to help identify and prevent problems. Unfortunately, knowledge about the condition, and particularly its prevalence, was overstated. The summary paper authored by Kimerly Yeager, Rosemary Agostini, Aurelia Nattiv, and Barbara Drinkwater noted, "Our understanding of this complex triad is unfortunately limited at this time."

Yet, in an effort to publicize the Triad, researchers and writers were not always careful to define the scope of the problem. In January 1994 *The Physician and Sportmedicine* magazine stated that "Young female athletes driven to excel in their chosen sports are at risk of developing a potentially fatal triad of disorders. By recognizing the connection between disordered eating, amenorrhea, and osteoporosis, physicians can help athletic young women stay active while avoiding significant morbidity."

In the two years following the ACSM conference, the Female Athlete Triad was a hot topic. At a national policy development forum on women's health issues in Washington, D.C., in 1994, the *only* presentation on health and fitness was devoted to the Female Athlete Triad. In an attempt to warn coaches, parents, and the health-care profession of a real problem, the media attention focused on the dramatic. What mother would encourage her daughter to become involved in sport that might lead to her death?

Carol Oglesby, a member of Melpomene's advisory board and a trustee of the Women's Sports Foundation, asked those writing and talking about the Triad to put it in context. She pointed out that the number of women suffering from the Triad is minuscule compared with the number of women who drop out of or never participate in sport as they move from adolescence to adulthood, yet this problem of nonparticipation doesn't seem to generate the kind of publicity in the mass media or calls from the scientific community for seminars, slide shows, and videos prompted by the Triad.

We agree with Oglesby that one of the major dangers is to label the series of disorders the Female Athlete Triad. She says, "The worst problem is the leap from the *few* studies of high-training athletes to a vague notion that 'all exercising women' need to look over their shoulder to see that the Triad is not lurking nearby." Although it is hard to document its extent, the Triad certainly also exists in the general population. Young athletes most at risk should be aware of the dangers, but we must not assume that it is limited to an athletic population.

These examples are but a few pointing to the need for more careful, judicious treatment of research findings in the popular press. We still have much to discover regarding women and exercise. Inaccurate reporting may discourage physical activity, and mistaken notions may lead women to sell their exercise bikes and hang up their running shoes. Mothers reading such information are forming opinions that may affect how readily they accept their daughter's interest in athletics.

Innuendos and distorted facts are powerful forces in our information society. Unfortunately, they have the power to discourage

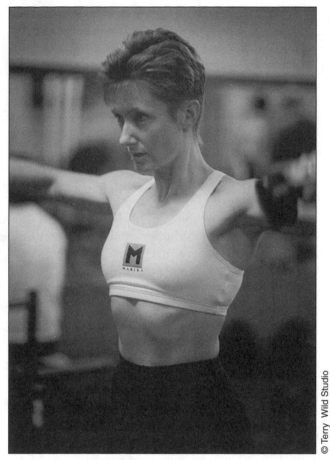

Health clubs now recruit women as well as men as members, stressing that exercise will improve their appearance as well as their health.

us from activities that could improve our health and change the very core of our beings.

To avoid being misled, we all need to listen more critically, ask more questions, and find out where we can go for information that we can trust. Throughout this book, we encourage you to walk completely around an issue until you see it from all sides. The latest reports are only a step in the process of understanding women and physical activity. They may or may not prove to be true as time goes by. With this in mind, we hope you'll listen to the "experts" with a grain of salt. Next time you hear someone say, "Stop exercising," consider the source, consider the times, and by all means, get a second opinion!

The Relationship Between Femininity and Sport

Ever since the Billie Jean King-Bobby Riggs match, it has been accept-able for women athletes to sweat. We now see positive images of strong, dedicated women athletes in the popular press, albeit concentrated for the most part in Olympic years. The image of the female athlete has even been used to sell commercial products, and female athletes now appear on Wheaties boxes.

On the other hand, it seems that society is still more comfortable with women who participate in sports that emphasize traditional feminine characteristics such as grace and beauty. We have all seen Olympic sportscasters make "sweethearts" out of gymnasts and figure skaters. Women in sports that require endurance or developed muscles are not so marketable. Where are the feature stories on women shot-putters or weight lifters? Indeed, strong women are somewhat suspect, and the Olympic gender testing requirement, for women only, is a particularly blatant example of this lingering suspicion. In a kind of compensatory behavior, many women in suspect sports go to great lengths to prove their femininity by wearing conspicuous jewelry or makeup on the playing field; some female basketball players even have "media con-sultants" to show them how to act and dress in ways considered to be traditionally feminine.

Homophobia

In the past 10 years a growing number of individuals in the women's sports movement have argued that concerns about femininity are a smoke screen for a far more complex and pervasive fear—homopho-bia, or the irrational fear of homosexuality. Indeed there are lesbians in women's sports just as there are in every segment of society, but the closet seems to be larger and murkier here and even harder to open than in other arenas of modern life.

As long as lesbianism is synonymous with shame, many lesbian women find that it is impossible to be open about their sexual orienta-tion. Consider, for instance, how damaging it is for a college coach to be accused of being a lesbian. Whether or not she is, and despite the irrel-evance of the question to her performance as a coach, she may lose the respect of fellow coaches. She often has a harder time recruiting ath-letes, and she may even lose influence with those who hold the purse strings. This threat alone is enough to force women into "apologetic" behaviors and, not incidentally, to keep men in a position of undue power.

Author Mariah Burton Nelson, who speaks openly of being lesbian, points out that labeling powerful women as lesbians is a time-honored tactic of those who wish to keep women in a secondary position. She believes we can end the lesbian stigma if women are open about their sexual orientation (whatever it is) and refuse to accept lesbianism as an epithet: "The only way to prevent gay-baiting from having any power is to be out, whether as lesbians or bisexual women or as advocates for lesbians or bisexual women. It doesn't work to say, 'oh, no, we're not lesbians.'"

Once again, we are called to disarm the myths so they cannot be used against us. Honest women such as Martina Navratilova prove to everyone that sexual orientation is not what's important about an athlete; sheer, miraculous talent is the focus.

Ageism

Not so many years ago few women beyond the age of 50 engaged in physical activity and sport. Women who look older, who have grey hair and bodies that show wrinkles and sags, are sometimes appalled and dismayed with response from the public. While we can see improvement, ageism is still alive and well. Rhoda, age 56, talks about running while on a business trip.

> "During the first half hour of my run, three men of varying ages made disparaging remarks to me; all of the remarks were related to my age. The first derogatory comment amused me. 'Hey, old bag,' a young man yelled, 'aren't you too old for that?' I cast a quick glance his way and surmised that his out-of-shape body would have trouble keeping up with my pace. But by the third time I was annoyed, and the comment took away some of the pleasure of the run."

We need to encourage, rather than discourage, physical activity. As recently as 1980 there were few separate age divisions in recreational events such as running or triathlons for women over 40. Now five-year age divisions go as high as 70. In 1995 Melpomene began awarding a special plaque to women over 80 who ran our 5K race. Women told us that even though the number of 70- and 80-year-olds who compete remains small, recognizing older athletes sent a powerful message.

Athletes With Disabilities

In the past, few women or men who had disabilities competed in sports. New acceptance and understanding of the possibilities that exist for those who often prefer to call themselves "differently abled" has encouraged the growth of these activities. One of the first sports to encourage wheelchair competition was road racing. In the 1970s, wheelchair divisions were added to such visible events as marathons; publicity encouraged others to try shorter distances. Wheelchair athletes now participate in tennis, basketball, swimming, archery, table tennis, squash, and racquetball. When the Paralympics are held in Atlanta in 1996, there will be 17 sports highlighting the skill and talent of athletes with disabilities. Linda Bunker, Dean of Students at the University of Virginia and a renowned psychologist, uses a wheelchair. She says:

> Wheelchair sports provide a unique opportunity for men and women to compete in the same sport. You learn that you can be better today than you were yesterday. I've found I can challenge myself by both subjective and objective standards. Participating in sports allows you to capitalize on your abilities rather than dwelling on what you can't do.

Larger Women

More attention is still needed to encourage the participation of larger women. Most do not fit the stereotype of what an athlete looks like. In addition they often have difficulty finding sportswear and equipment that is correctly sized. Clearly there is a need to expand the image of who an athlete is and what she looks like.

WHAT LIES AHEAD?

It's hard to know what the future may hold. If the past decade predicts a fast pace of change in societal attitudes and expectations, we can expect far more girls and women to participate in physical activity. Since Melpomene's founding in 1982, attitudes about what is appropriate for women have shown some dramatic changes. In that year, 25 percent of the respondents to our first membership study told us that societal expectations were an obstacle to physical activity. They specifically said, "people believing I shouldn't be athletic" deterred them from physical activity. Just 8 years later, only 6 percent cited that as an obstacle. Similarly, fear of not doing well was cited by 29 percent of the respondents in 1982 but by only 9 percent in 1990. Lack of encouragement was cited as an obstacle by 27 percent in 1982 and by only 7 percent in 1990. According to officials at the National Federation of State High School Associations, the number of girls participating in sports at the high school level rose in 1993-94 for the fifth consecutive year to 2,130,315. In Minnesota, closer attention to gender equity resulted in adding ice hockey as a high school girls' sport. In 1994, the first year, 24 teams were organized. In 1995, 49 girls' teams hit the ice.

It's clear that girls and women of all sizes, ages, and abilities are beginning to get the message that it's fun to be physically active.

SUMMARY

In this chapter we've shared stories of progress and change. We've also pointed out that problems and challenges remain. In the following chapters we'll share more research and stories that will make it easier for you to incorporate physical activity into your own lives. Many women tell us at Melpomene that taking up cross-country skiing, walking, or biking is the best thing they've done for their own personal sense of well-being. Says Mary Lou: "I feel much stronger, and I'm much more confident about the way I look. But the real plus of physical activity is that I take time for myself on a daily basis. That makes me a better mother, partner, and friend. I'd recommend it to anyone!"

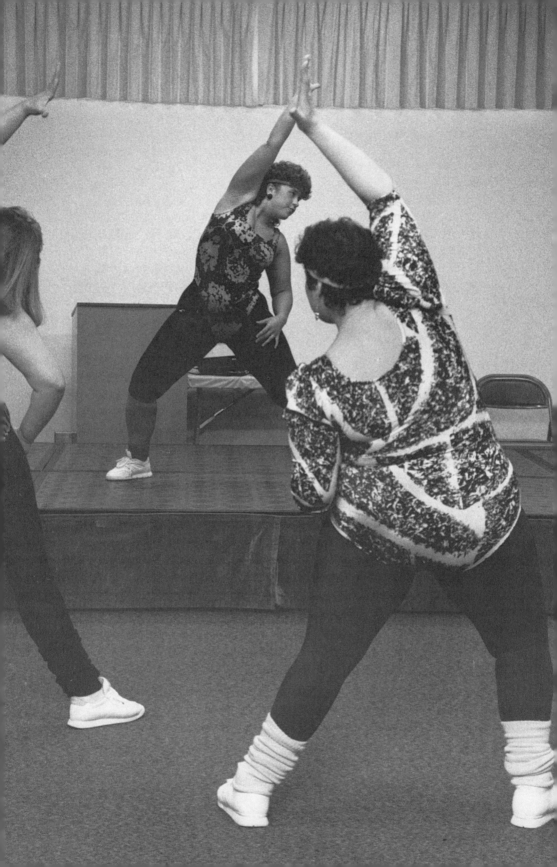

2

What Do You See in Your Mirror?

Lisa is a 46-year-old mother who's feeling particularly fat and frumpy one morning. When her 17-year-old daughter says, "Mom, you look really pretty," Lisa sarcastically rolls her eyes. "Mom, I'm serious," her daughter says. "Why do you believe me when I tell you something doesn't look good, but always think I'm kidding when I honestly try to compliment you? I think you need some help with your body image."

"I've learned to be very happy in a body that is 5 feet, 8 inches, and weighs 240 pounds," says Pat. "I've maintained that weight for the past 20 years and know it is a healthy weight for me. Yet, I also know people still make value judgments because they assume I can change my body size."

Body image is the picture of our physical selves that we carry in our mind's eye. Often, this image has little resemblance to how we actually look. Our attitudes, perceptions, and value judgments overlay the mental picture, giving us an emotional rather than an objective view.

How accurate is your body image? Is it possible to change the way you feel about your body? In this chapter, we'll introduce you to some of the latest research into body image and help you sort out what is truthful and what is unrealistic about your own body image. We'll also look at the prejudices and beliefs that many of us have about different body shapes, and see how these perceptions can wound self-esteem. Finally, we'll investigate ways that you can reject certain unrealistic ideals and learn to love the body you have.

Before you read the chapter, you may want to check out some of your current beliefs by taking the quiz on page 33. The questions reflect both opinions and facts. The test will not be scored, because there are no right or wrong answers to the opinion questions. Instead, your answers will serve to document what you currently believe about body image. After you finish the chapter, take the test again to see if your perception has changed.

Body image—how you perceive your physical self—is a complex part of your self-image that begins to form in infancy and evolves throughout life. Your idea of your body is a composite of the attitudes of your parents, your classmates, and later, your adult peers. The attitudes of those around you are usually reflections of how the society at large views different body shapes. It's difficult not to internalize the images of women that surround you every day in magazines and on television.

WHEN DO WE DEVELOP OUR BODY IMAGE?

Stop and reflect on your own body image. When were you first aware of how you looked? Chances are you were aware of your body image even before you knew how you felt about yourself as a person. You may have noticed that your body had an impact on the way people looked at you and treated you.

What Do You Believe?

	Agree	Neutral	Disagree
If you have ever been fat, it is very difficult to lose a "fat body" image.	☐	☐	☐
It is possible to be too thin.	☐	☐	☐
Body fat measurements are the best indicators of fitness and fatness.	☐	☐	☐
An ideal body fat percentage for a 40-year-old woman is 19 percent.	☐	☐	☐
Women's perceptions of their bodies are often inaccurate.	☐	☐	☐
The media are responsible for an increased number of eating disorders.	☐	☐	☐
Women are constantly encouraged to make changes in their appearance.	☐	☐	☐
Thin women are more likely to attract men and get better jobs.	☐	☐	☐
Athletes who are thin perform better than those who are heavier.	☐	☐	☐
Preschool children choose thin playmates over fatter ones.	☐	☐	☐
By the time girls are in high school, they are more likely than boys to be dissatisfied with their body shape.	☐	☐	☐
High school girls of average weight are more likely to go to college than girls who are obese.	☐	☐	☐
Men like women fatter than we think they do.	☐	☐	☐
I feel better about my body than I did five years ago.	☐	☐	☐
I could never be too thin.	☐	☐	☐
I have favorable memories of the way I looked as a child.	☐	☐	☐
I constantly worry about my weight or my eating patterns.	☐	☐	☐
Friends are more important to me than the way I look.	☐	☐	☐

Body Image During Childhood

What other people say makes a difference at a very early age. Body image for girls is much more problematic than for boys. Many of the early messages you receive are already very gender based. Perhaps you remember getting messages like this as a little girl: "Aren't you pretty" or "You're lucky you're so petite!" Few women have favorable memories of hearing, "My, how strong you are," or "You're going to be big and tall." Those were usually reserved for little boys. Somehow, even at a young age, we got the message that it was not flattering to be called "strong" or to have too much athletic prowess.

How did these early messages affect how we would feel about our bodies as adults? Few studies address the complex issues of how body image is formed, and how physical activity as a child might affect that perception. Melpomene researcher Vicki Novak Johnson conducted a study in the late eighties that looked at the socialization patterns of children at early ages. We were interested in finding out what impact, if any, a mother's exercise history might have on how she socializes her child.

Results indicated that mothers who were more physically active were more likely to describe their children in terms of skills and personality rather than by body shape and size. Unfortunately, this runs counter to the norm. Most people emphasize body shape and size when describing children, and as a result youngsters become aware of being fat or thin at a very early age. Studies show that by preschool, boys and girls are already choosing thin children as playmates over fatter ones, with obvious implications for self-esteem. Fat children need positive messages that they are "OK" the way they are so they can learn to accept themselves and ignore societal pressures to be thin.

In a classic study conducted in Montreal by psychologists Beverly Katz Mendelson and Donna Romano White, 36 subjects aged 7.5 to 12 years old completed a self-esteem and body-esteem questionnaire. Sixteen of the subjects—11 girls and 5 boys—were more than 15 percent overweight. These children had a lower opinion of their bodies and personal appearance than children of average weight, suggesting that they had already accepted the cultural norm that says thinner is better. The authors also found that "Children who are dissatisfied with personal appearances are also dissatisfied with aspects of their lives unrelated to looks, aspects such as intellectual and school status, behavior, and anxiety." The overweight children did not yet suffer from lower self-esteem, however. They were still able to say, "I don't like my body very well, but I like myself." In subsequent studies with more subjects, Mendelson and White found that this level of self-esteem doesn't last very long. By later adolescence, overweight girls were much more likely than normal-weight girls to develop low self-esteem related to body size.

Another interesting study of 406 children enrolled in grades four to six in a midwestern community was conducted by Susan Ferencz Stager and Peter Burke. In this study, both girls and boys used the same terms to describe fat children, including "less good looking," "more often teased," and "having fewer friends." Some children saw themselves in the fat child stereotype, even if they were not overweight. The children who identified most strongly with the fat child stereotype had the lowest self-esteem. Stager and Burke also found that the skinny child stereotype was viewed favorably. In fact, when compared with a study done 10 years earlier, the skinny child stereotype had become even more favorable.

Because the negative consequences of being overweight seem only to get worse as a child gets older, Carol Johnson of Largely Positive, Inc., stresses the importance of building self-esteem in larger kids at a young age. In a 1993 article in *Obesity and Health*, Johnson emphasizes the need for parents to accept their own bodies instead of criticizing them all the time. By doing this, you become a strong, positive role model for your child. Johnson also advises parents not to put children on a diet. Concentrating on healthy eating and encouraging children to find some form of physical activity they enjoy is a much more positive approach. She also says to praise larger children for their accomplishments and talents so they will learn that self-worth is not related to weight and that they are just as good as thinner kids. Finally, Johnson says, it's important that they know that greater weight doesn't make them less attractive than thinner children and that you love them unconditionally. Following these suggestions can help larger kids learn to love and accept themselves.

Pressures Increase in High School

If the growing number of weight-conscious children in grade school disturbs you, wait until you hear the statistics on those in high school! By high school, the obsession with weight and dieting becomes extremely common, especially among girls. The Youth Risk Behavior Study, conducted in 1989 and 1990 with 11,467 high school students, found that 44 percent of the female students were trying to lose weight. An additional 26 percent were trying to keep from gaining weight. In the 1988 National Adolescent and School Health Survey of 8th- and

10th-grade students, 61 percent of girls reported dieting during the past year. Direct comparison of the two studies is difficult because one asks generally about trying to lose weight and the other specifically talks about dieting, but the message is clear: High school girls are worried about weight. In comparison, 15 percent of boys were trying to lose weight, and 28 percent reported dieting during the past year. The 1994 *Glamour* "Daughters of Dieters" study found that 58 percent of girls said their parents were critical of their weight in high school, and 72 percent reported being on a diet.

It's important to note that the statistics for black girls differed in the Youth Risk Behavior Study. A 1989 paper in the *Journal of School Health* by Sharon Desmond, James Price, and colleagues found that black adolescents have a significantly higher rate of satisfaction with their appearances than white adolescents. The authors suggest a possible explanation is that black adolescents may have different ideas of beauty that aren't based on being thin. Melpomene's 1994 study with girls involved in YWCA summer programs nationwide supports that hypothesis. Forty-one percent of white girls worried about weight, as compared with 31 percent of African American respondents. Likewise,

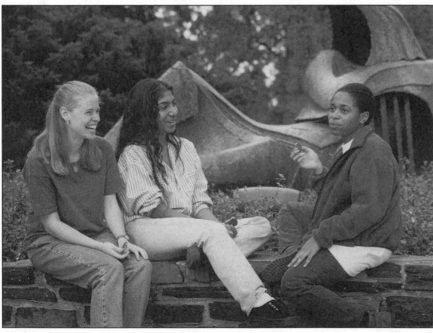

Perhaps no one is more self-conscious and body-aware than high school girls in the United States.

50 percent of black girls "liked the way they looked," as compared with only 21 percent of white girls.

Boys don't seem nearly as dissatisfied with body shape as girls are. In a late 1980s Gallup poll, 59 percent of teenage girls said they wanted to lose weight, compared with only 20 percent of the boys. For girls, this perceived need to lose weight might be related to the natural changes of puberty. Many girls feel that the onset of menstruation and the swelling of their breasts is something that simply happens to them; though they may worry about the timing of these events, there's not much they can do to control them. To a great extent, additional weight is also part of maturing, but girls seem to view it differently. Along with the rest of society, they see body weight as something that a disciplined person should be able to manipulate and control. Perhaps weight control steals center stage because this is the one area where adolescent girls feel they can influence their bodies.

The shape many girls are striving for is often not a healthy one. The aforementioned Gallup poll showed that girls who were asked to choose their ideal weight inevitably chose one that was at least 10 percent below the recommended "ideal" weight. All the girls, whether they were within recommended ranges or not, described themselves as being overweight. This tendency to define oneself as fatter than is objectively true persists throughout most of a woman's life.

A woman's perception of her own body is often based on what she thinks someone else finds attractive. A need to conform and therefore be accepted may be most important during high school and college years. In a survey of 500 college-aged men and women, Paul Rozin and April Fallon of the University of Pennsylvania found that women say they are heavier than what they think men find attractive. Moreover, they would prefer to weigh even less than the ideal body weight they think men would choose. Are these women seeking the media stereotype of anorexic thinness? Interestingly, when men were questioned, they said that they actually liked somewhat heavier women. In other studies in which men and women were asked to identify attractive body sizes, the men viewed a greater range of weights as potentially attractive. They were also more tolerant of their own excess weight than the women were.

HOW SOCIETY SHAPES OUR BODY IMAGE

In some societies, a large, rounded woman is viewed as being a fertile woman and is therefore admired. Today, in our largely overfed culture, many Americans are gripped by a feverish obsession to be thin and fit. Thinness is associated with high social class, with success, and with the ability to attract a man. The standard of white female beauty has become more narrowly defined and restrictive, making it nearly impossible to be thin enough, fit enough, or young enough. Society, in effect, keeps moving the finish line farther and farther back, ensuring that most of us will never attain the unrealistic "ideal."

Psychologist Bean Robinson, PhD, writing in the February 1985 *Melpomene Report,* reminds us that "thinness has not always been viewed with such universal fervor and longing. In earlier times, from approximately 1400-1900, the more voluptuous abundant female figure was seen as the ideal type."

Western taste keeps changing, giving us at least three different ideal body types for women since about 1500. The first was tummy-centered and often quite fat. William Bennet and Joel Gurin, authors of the book *The Dieter's Dilemma—Eating Less and Weighing More,* call her the "reproductive figure." Between 1650 and 1700, taste changed throughout Europe to a new ideal which was rather plump and all bosom and bottom; her narrow, often-corseted waist was designed to emphasize these ample endowments. Bennet and Gurin label this type the "maternal figure." Then, rather rapidly between 1910 and 1920, this full-blown female figure lost favor within Anglo-American culture and was replaced by a tubular, lean, and slender figure with minimal breasts and buttocks and little remnant of the promising, reproductive tummy. Bennet and Gurin call her the "sexual free agent." Now the emphasis is sexuality which may or may not be related to reproduction.

While there has been some fluctuation of ideal body weight and shape in the twentieth century, the general trend has been toward even thinner models. A 1930s magazine titled *Fitness,* which includes several articles devoted to women and physical fitness, portrays healthy women who are clearly 20 pounds heavier than those we would find in a 1996 publication. Today, even magazines devoted to skiing, running, tennis, or cycling all use models for their covers who look as if they are on an 800-calorie-a-day diet. The *Playboy* centerfold has lost 25 pounds in the last 20 years. She is now 18 percent thinner than what is considered the medical ideal or normal for her age and height. In a short span of time, we have moved from at least a gently rounded figure to the woman whom nutritionist Julie Jones, PhD, describes as "the backless, frontless, buttless wonder."

This ideal body image doesn't necessarily hold true for women with different cultural backgrounds. As noted earlier, some research, mostly on girls, suggests that African Americans don't ascribe to the same beauty ideal as white women. A 1990 study by Regina Casper and Daniel Offer found that black female adolescents were less concerned about dieting and gaining weight than white female adolescents. According to a 1994 study by Mimi Nichter and colleagues, the ideal body image for black women has more to do with accepting one's own body and having a personal sense of style. Personality is also an important part of overall attractiveness. Black girls have higher self-esteem than white girls because, unlike white girls, they tend not to compare themselves with a single physical ideal.

Our National Obsession With Thinness

As women, we are constantly encouraged to work toward a lean, tubular shape, even though it may be structurally impossible or even medically dangerous for us to be so skinny. Losing weight has become synonymous with "taking care of yourself," or "not letting yourself go." Next time you are in the checkout line at the supermarket, scan the headline articles of leading women's magazines. Notice how many magazines have a "makeover" that stresses weight loss. Almost all of these magazines feature dieting articles every month except December, when they emphasize the psychological importance of food! Further, our obsession seems to be growing. Writing for *Nutrition Today*, authors Dorice Czajka-Narins and Ellen Parnham note that in the years between 1950 and 1983, the number of articles in five popular women's magazines about dieting and losing weight increased while the weight of models decreased.

At Melpomene, we're concerned about the impact of this trend on young women. In 1991 Elissa Koff and Jill Rierdan surveyed 206 sixth-grade girls on weight, body image, dieting practices, and attitudes toward weight and eating. Their results suggest that "feeling too fat and wishing to lose weight were becoming normative for young adolescent girls in that the majority of girls wished to weigh less and said that they dieted at least occasionally." Fifty-three percent of the girls said they had dieted; for 70 percent of the girls concerns about weight emerged between ages 9 and 11. The authors also say "what is perhaps most striking about these data is the pervasiveness of embracing a diet mentality even among girls who did not perceive themselves to be overweight and who were not dissatisfied with how they looked at their current weight."

WHAT IT MEANS TO BE LARGE

The terminology often used in referring to body size is laden with judgment. In her book *Great Shape,* Pat Lyons describes the difficulty of finding a term for size that is accurate without being demeaning. The medical profession uses the term obese, and you'll find us using that term occasionally in this book. It isn't our preference, however, because it implies disease. According to Lyons, the term "overweight" is commonly used by people trying to be polite, but it implies that there is a lower weight to which fat people should conform. Until we understand the physiological processes underlying the maintenance of body size, using the term overweight just raises the question, 'over *what* weight?'" Lyons concludes that *fat* is the best word to use but says that until that term is commonly used in a matter-of-fact way the word *large* is preferable.

The Consequences of Being Large

In a society in which thinness is rewarded, being large can be both a social and an economic liability. A large person is often seen as being out of control and socially undesirable. Large people are frequently described as "lazy," "awkward," "weak willed," and "dumb."

To understand what motivates this destructive behavior, think about what it means to be thin in America. "You can never be too rich or too thin," the saying goes. And indeed, thinness seems to be equated with material success and happiness.

A 1993 study in the *New England Journal of Medicine* conducted by Steven Gortmaker, Aviva Must, and colleagues seems to confirm your suspicion. They studied a large number of women and men at two points during a 7-year period. They concluded that "being overweight during adolescence has important social and economic consequences which are greater than those of many other chronic physical conditions." Women who were overweight had completed fewer years of school, were less likely to be married, and had household incomes that were $6,710 per year lower, *independent* of baseline socioeconomic status and aptitude test scores. Gortmaker further states that "discrimination against people who are overweight may account for these results."

Knowing that body shape can have such an enormous impact, is it really shocking or surprising that some young mothers start their children on diets when they are only 6 months old? "Daughters of Dieters," a 1994 *Glamour* article by Anne Taylor Fleming, discusses a survey by *Glamour* that examined the effect of parents' eating habits on their children. They found that girls internalize their parents' attitudes about food, diets, and body image at a very young age. These attitudes form a lasting impression that carries into adulthood. Sixty percent of the 4,000 women polled had memories of their mothers dieting. They reported becoming aware of their mothers' efforts to "slim down" at age 10.

G. Terrance Wilson, a professor of psychology at Rutgers University, says that "no matter how 'perfect' a woman's figure may be, if she is told she looks fat, she will have an emotional reaction out of proportion to reality. On the other hand, if you tell her she looks thin or has lost weight, she will be inordinately pleased." Think about it: How often have you told someone that she looks fat?

Several women were discussing this issue at a Melpomene conference. One woman remarked: "Only once did anyone tell me I looked fat. I was devastated, even though I knew it was not objectively true. I had gained about 10 pounds and dreaded having someone say I looked heavier. Most of my friends are sensitive to the fact that I struggle with a distorted fat body image and have a tendency to think that thin is better. They would probably never tell me I looked heavier because they would know I would have the reaction Wilson describes."

The ironic fact is that this woman had been a very thin runner and actually looked better at her new weight. Perhaps her deep-seated fear of being fat kept her from seeing the true image of herself in the mirror. Like most of us, she was programmed to believe that any weight gain, even if it is needed, is a dangerous trend.

The Truth About Size

Brownell's excellent paper "Understanding and Treating Obesity" suggests that we need to look carefully at the studies linking obesity with health problems. Media "experts" and many physicians would have us believe that even 10 extra pounds will make us more susceptible to long-term health problems. Granted, there may be health risks related to obesity, but it is not clear that weight per se should always be blamed for medical problems that a large person may encounter. In fact, Brownell states that the worst dangers of obesity may not be physical in nature, but rather, "the psychological and social hazards of obesity may be as serious as the medical hazards."

A popular myth is that large people could be thin if only they were physically active. This argument loses steam when you think about the thin people you know who aren't active at all. Why is it that they are able to eat all they want, live a sedentary lifestyle, and yet not become fat? Why don't fat people who exercise regularly become thin? Mounting evidence seems to indicate that the difference between fat people and thin people is not in their eating or their activity patterns but rather in their biological makeup.

Large people are often blamed for creating their own condition through gluttony or a simple lack of self-control. The fact is that many large people are very conscious of controlling their intake of calories. Evidence reveals that even at similar intakes, large people face greater odds than people of average weight when they try to lose weight.

Each person has her own unique metabolism; every body burns fuel differently. Researchers have also found that the amount of energy (or food) that a body needs in order to function at a given weight varies from person to person. After reviewing the literature related to caloric intake and weight, Sue Dyrenforth, Orland Wooley, and Susan Wooley concluded that "some women gain on 5,000 calories per day, some gain on 800." This means that two people can both be sitting and watching TV, but one will burn more calories per hour than the other simply by virtue of a faster metabolism. The greatest documented difference was 770 calories.

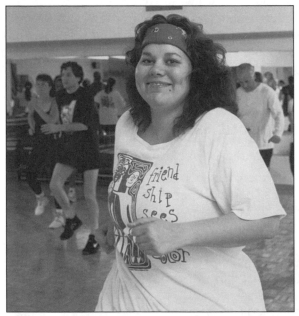

© David R. Barnes

Your metabolism—the way your body burns fuel—
is as individual as you are.

Why do these differences occur? It is only recently that we have begun to examine the role of heredity in relation to weight. In December 1994, Dr. Jeffrey Friedman and colleagues at Rockefeller University in New York City reported the isolation of a gene that may be linked to obesity in mice. This gene, named the ob gene, produces a protein that tells the part of the brain that controls appetite when to reduce or increase food intake. In some people, the part of the brain that controls appetite will think the body doesn't have enough fat and will signal the intake of more food than is necessary. Further research is currently under way to discover if this is true for humans.

The link with heredity had already been established by Albert Stunkard, Terryl Foch, and Hrubec Zdenek, who analyzed data collected from a large number of twins and concluded that "human fatness is under strong genetic control." Stunkard has also done research that found that adopted children had body weights that were more closely matched with their biological parents than with their adoptive parents. Maybe the old adage that says we should look at our mothers to see how we will age has more truth to it than we would like to admit!

As hard as it may be to accept, the fact is that we don't have a great deal of choice about the shape of our bodies. Ellen Goodman, syndicated columnist, has a novel approach to the problem. She suggests that we all grow several inches in the next year! We've considered offering a height-raising clinic at Melpomene; certainly if one can manipulate weight, height should also be susceptible to change! We immediately see how ridiculous this idea is, yet for many women, it's just as impossible to hope that they will one day wear a size 9 or 11.

What if you are fat? For many women, being large is a fact of life. An estimated 16 million women in America wear size 16 or larger and therefore are labeled large or fat by society. One of these women, Alice Ansfield, who has a master's degree in clinical psychology, was tired of fighting prejudice and isolation; she was tired of focusing energy on the desire to be thin. In 1984 she decided to produce a positive, life-giving publication for large women like herself. *Radiance: The Magazine for Large Women* features articles and stories "from women of all walks of life who have become experts on their own experiences as large women living in an anti-fat world." The focus is on good health and positive self-esteem, a much needed but hard-to-achieve commodity for many large women.

In an article written for the Winter 1988 *Melpomene* journal, Ansfield (*Radiance* editor) and Pat Lyons report that discrimination and human isolation extract a heavy toll in the lives of most large women:

Rather than be encouraged to inhabit the world as strong, healthy, vital people, many women of all sizes live instead in perpetual terror of gaining weight and measure their entire self-worth by the numbers on the scale. They postpone education, social life, creativity, career, and involvement in community activities, putting their energies instead into efforts to achieve an elusive, magical point in the future defined as 'when I am thin.' That many never reach that stage is a tragic story of wasted lives.

Of course, many women who are not technically fat are also held hostage by their preoccupation with weight; studies reveal that 60 to 80 percent of adult American women have this concern.

Your Perceptions of Large Women

Do you find that you are more critical of people who are fat? Are you more critical of fat women than fat men? Earlier, we described some of the myths and negative attitudes that stifle large women. We also showed you evidence that fat women generally do not overeat, and that for some women, being thin will never be a realistic or a healthy option. Even with this new knowledge, you still may be forming judgments based on old stereotypes. One way to test your sensitivity and perhaps reverse your judgments is to take the following test.

Robinson's Fat Phobia Scale—The "F-Scale"

Listed below are adjectives sometimes used to describe obese or fat people. Please indicate your beliefs about what fat people are like on the following items by placing an X on the line that best describes your feelings and beliefs.

1. lazy — — — — — industrious
2. sloppy — — — — — neat
3. disgusting — — — — — not disgusting
4. friendly — — — — — unfriendly
5. nonassertive — — — — — assertive
6. no willpower — — — — — has willpower
7. artistic — — — — — not artistic
8. creative — — — — — uncreative
9. warm — — — — — cold
10. depressed — — — — — happy
11. smart — — — — — stupid
12. reads a lot — — — — — doesn't read a lot
13. unambitious — — — — — ambitious
14. easy to talk to — — — — — hard to talk to
15. unattractive — — — — — attractive
16. miserable — — — — — jolly
17. selfish — — — — — selfless

18. poor self-control	__ __ __ __ __	good self-control
19. inconsiderate of others	__ __ __ __ __	considerate of others
20. good	__ __ __ __ __	bad
21. popular	__ __ __ __ __	unpopular
22. important	__ __ __ __ __	insignificant
23. slow	__ __ __ __ __	fast
24. ineffective	__ __ __ __ __	effective
25. careless	__ __ __ __ __	careful
26. having endurance	__ __ __ __ __	having no endurance
27. inactive	__ __ __ __ __	active
28. nice complexion	__ __ __ __ __	bad complexion
29. tries to please people	__ __ __ __ __	doesn't try to please people
30. humorous/funny	__ __ __ __ __	humorless/not funny
31. inefficient	__ __ __ __ __	efficient
32. strong	__ __ __ __ __	weak
33. individualistic	__ __ __ __ __	not individualistic
34. pitiful	__ __ __ __ __	not pitiful
35. independent	__ __ __ __ __	dependent
36. good-natured	__ __ __ __ __	irritable
37. self-indulgent	__ __ __ __ __	self-sacrificing
38. passive	__ __ __ __ __	aggressive
39. indirect	__ __ __ __ __	direct
40. likes food	__ __ __ __ __	dislikes food
41. dirty	__ __ __ __ __	clean
42. does not attend to own appearance	__ __ __ __ __	very attentive to own appearance
43. easygoing	__ __ __ __ __	uptight
44. shapeless	__ __ __ __ __	shapely
45. overeats	__ __ __ __ __	undereats
46. smells bad	__ __ __ __ __	smells good
47. sweaty	__ __ __ __ __	not sweaty
48. moody	__ __ __ __ __	even-tempered
49. insecure	__ __ __ __ __	secure
50. low self-esteem	__ __ __ __ __	high self-esteem

Reprinted by permission from B. Robinson, 1985, "The Stigma of Obesity: Fat Fallacies Debunked," *Melpomene Report* 4(1):9-13.

Psychologist Beatrice "Bean" Robinson, the author of the Fat Phobia Scale (F-Scale), reports that a majority of the 856 people who filled out her questionnaire chose more negative than positive adjectives when asked to describe their feelings and beliefs about fat people. The data show that people do indeed harbor a strong negative stereotype about fat people.

Some of the more common negative comments were that fat people like food, overeat, have low self-esteem, and are insecure, shapeless, and inactive. Respondents also had some positive things to say about fat people, however, commenting that they were friendly, warm, easy to talk to, and humorous.

Robinson administers the Fat Phobia Scale to her fat clients before and after they go through a program created by Robinson and her colleague, psychologist Jane Bacon. The program is designed to improve the self-esteem and body image of people who are at least 50 pounds over their recommended weight. The majority of these clients say they have more positive attitudes toward fat people after completing the program. This suggests that fat phobia, which Robinson describes as a fear and hatred of fat people, can be changed by education and group therapy.

If you aren't a large woman, but are critical of those who are, and fearful of becoming fat yourself, this may be the time to try to change those attitudes. It may not be easy.

"The *Melpomene* journal article on 'Fat Phobia' was interesting," remarked a Melpomene volunteer several years ago. "I know I have a prejudice against fat people; I'm always sure they can control their weight!" Having believed that for 58 years, this woman continues to relate stories and experiences that are helping her slowly change her opinions. Fat women are beginning to speak out about their experiences; many are developing self-images that allow them to be secure with who they are. Clothing manufacturers such as Full Bloom and Fit to be Tried, and magazines such as *Radiance* play a big part in helping these women make that change.

We do not all have the same opportunity to be thin adults. Psychologist Albert Stunkard says that families who have a history of obesity "will really have to work on trying to prevent obesity in their kids." Once these children are adults, they too are going to have to "remain eternally vigilant against gaining weight." Stunkard and his colleagues conclude that the struggle is worth it because of the emotional and physical problems of being overweight.

Do you agree? There are certainly societal disadvantages to being fat. Yet many women, after years of unsuccessful dieting, regret all the time they've wasted worrying about gaining weight. They are eager to explore new ideas and approaches to weight and body image; they want to work on accepting the bodies that they have. Flying in the face of everything society believes about body size, women of all weights are beginning to build foundations of self-respect. Conferences or small groups facilitated by a clinical psychologist are offered in some areas to help women readjust their body images. Some foresighted educators are working with young women before the lifetime patterns of self-loathing become too deeply ingrained.

An ideal age during which to work on these concepts is the high school years. Leslie McBride, a professor in the school of health and physical education at Portland State University, has worked with adolescents in a group situation designed to get them to look more objectively and positively at themselves. She asks them to make two lists; one enumerates positive physical features about one's self, the other negative features. Next, cards with the names of each participant are distributed. The group is then instructed to write down a positive comment about the physical appearance of the person whose name appears on the top of the card.

Imagine the results. Many students reported that they had never really thought about themselves as they were described by others. Being told that you have particularly beautiful eyes, that you look strong, or that your smile always encourages others has a positive influence that can affect the way you feel about your body.

A similar exercise would be a good starting place for adults trying to work on body image issues. Try a simple test. Ask any friend about her best physical features; she will probably hesitate at first and often not even be aware of something that others find particularly attractive or outstanding.

Janette's hair started to turn gray long before many of her friends' hair. After several years of fooling around with coloring, she decided it wasn't worth the effort. Suddenly people started complimenting her on her beautiful hair, which to this day surprises her. Janette's experience reminds us that the image we have of ourselves may be worlds different from how others see us. Learning to accept and believe genuine compliments may help you start to change your inner picture of yourself.

It's important to remember that you are creating impressions for the younger women in your life. In 1993 Jane Helmke, a producer at KARE 11 TV, a Minnesota-based Gannett affiliate, created an hour-long special, "Heroes, Growing up Female and Strong," that showed women of many shapes, sizes, and ethnic backgrounds who were happy with their bodies. Thousands of girls nationwide have viewed the video. Many tell us it helps them realize that physical beauty does not have to be defined as blond and thin.

HOW ACCURATE IS YOUR BODY IMAGE?

Clearly, many of our attitudes about our bodies are formed when we are younger, and are further defined by what we think is appropriate or expected of us. There seems to be a separate set of expectations for men and women, and evidence of cultural differences is growing as well. An Asian Melpomene staff member told us that body image issues were primarily based on how she is perceived in a predominantly white society: "Many Asian women don't worry about weight or other typically white issues as much as they worry about looking different." This correlates to evidence that African American girls do not seem to be as concerned with weight issues.

How Do You Perceive Your Weight?

To examine your current feelings, try the following exercise: Look at the pictures presented below and choose the one you think best reflects your body size. Now select the body size you would like to have. Are they the same?

Five Body Sizes—Which One Is You?

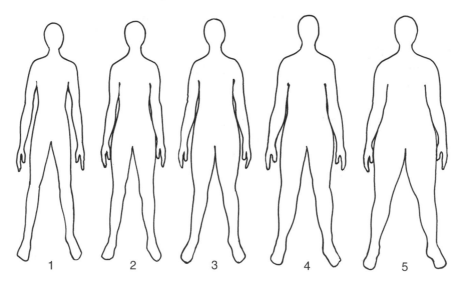

The drawings above represent bodies that are (1) 20 percent underweight, (2) 10 percent underweight, (3) of average weight, (4) 10 percent overweight, and (5) 20 percent overweight. If you chose one of the underweight figures for your "ideal," you are not alone. In 1984, we asked physically active women whose average age was 32 to do just what you did. Thirty-eight percent of the respondents said they would like to be 20 percent underweight and an additional 44 percent said they would like to be 10 percent underweight. Only 14 percent thought that an average size body was desirable!

In 1994, we repeated the study with a group of women representing a wider range of physical activity. These women, participants at the National Rural Electric Cooperative Association Executive Secretaries' national convention, were even more likely than those surveyed in 1984 to select thin figures as the ideal body type. Forty-four percent chose the 20 percent underweight figure, and another 44 percent chose the figure that is 10 percent underweight. Only 11 percent of the women, whose average age was 43, chose the average size body. When we compared desired body size with the size they believed themselves to be, 36 percent wanted to be one body shape smaller, and 45 percent wanted to be two shapes smaller. On observation, the women were thin-appearing, yet 81 percent wanted to be even smaller! In both cases, the sample was 95 percent white; new evidence suggests the results would be different if the majority of respondents were black.

In a similar study of college-age women, researchers Miller, Coffman, and Linke found that 63 percent of the women overestimated their own size. The desired weight for women in the study was 116 pounds, or 14 pounds less than their reported weight. Look again at the silhouettes. Did you say you wanted a body that is 10 percent underweight? How accurate do you think you are in assessing your true body shape? To test your self-perception, ask both a male and a female friend to select the body shape most like yours.

Here's another question. Do you consider yourself underweight, slightly underweight, just right, slightly overweight, or overweight? Don't be surprised if you chose one of the overweight categories. Melpomene Institute has conducted three membership studies—one in 1982, a second in 1985, and a third in 1990. As shown on page 50, the percentage of women who consider themselves "just right" has improved slightly over the years. However, when we surveyed midlife women, ranging in age from 40 to 66 in 1993, 56 percent reported they were overweight to some degree, yet when we compared their weights with the 1991 USDA chart of acceptable weights, we found that 97 percent of those who considered themselves slightly overweight were inaccurate. Their weights were actually within the "acceptable" range.

If you chose a small body size which may not be healthy for you personally, this might be the time to start looking at the issue more realistically. If you are 5 feet, 4 inches, weigh 130 pounds, and are among those who would "give anything" to lose 10 pounds, consider the possibility that the effort required to lose it may not bring the desired results. Many experts agree that losing or gaining 5-10 pounds does not make much difference in appearance or health status. If, on the other hand, you weigh 200 pounds, a change in eating and exercise habits that results in a 10- to 20-pound weight loss could actually improve your health status, at least in the short term. Diabetes, hypertension, and blood cholesterol seem particularly sensitive to change.

Weight Perceptions of Melpomene Members

Responses to the question "Do you consider yourself . . . ?

	1982	1985	1990
Underweight	1.0%	.5%	.4%
Slightly underweight	1.5	3.1	3.9
Just right	37.1	39.7	41.7
Slightly overweight	52.8	47.8	44.0
Overweight	7.6	8.9	9.2

Which Parts Do You Like Best?

Dissatisfaction with your body is not always related to weight. The way you feel about your body as a whole may be related to how you feel about various parts of your body. Rating your arms, legs, face, and so forth in the questionnaire on page 51 may help you identify areas of satisfaction or concern.

Your peer group and social environment may also have something to do with your level of satisfaction. A 1994 Melpomene study of girls who attended YWCA summer programs confirms earlier research conducted by Sharon Desmond and Mimi Nichter suggesting that black and white girls use different measures to define attractiveness. Weight in particular seems less problematic for black girls. Thirty-two percent of black girls reported worrying about weight "too much" as compared with 41 percent of white girls. While these differences are not earth-shattering, the fact that 40 percent of black girls consider themselves attractive or very attractive as compared with 9 percent of white girls shows a clear difference. Black girls were also much less likely to compare themselves to other girls. Forty-four percent of black girls in the Melpomene study had a high body image as compared with 31.8 percent of white girls.

Body Parts Questionnaire

	Have strong negative feelings and wish change could somehow be made	Don't like but can put up with	Have no particular feelings one way or the other	Am satisfied	Consider myself fortunate
1. Hair	1	2	3	4	5
2. Teeth	1	2	3	4	5
3. Eyes	1	2	3	4	5
4. Ears	1	2	3	4	5
5. Nose	1	2	3	4	5
6. Skin	1	2	3	4	5
7. Overall facial attractiveness	1	2	3	4	5
8. Arms	1	2	3	4	5
9. Breasts/chest	1	2	3	4	5
10. Shoulders	1	2	3	4	5
11. Abdomen	1	2	3	4	5
12. Hips	1	2	3	4	5
13. Waist	1	2	3	4	5
14. Upper legs (thighs)	1	2	3	4	5
15. Lower legs (calves)	1	2	3	4	5
16. Body build	1	2	3	4	5
17. Posture	1	2	3	4	5
18. Weight	1	2	3	4	5
19. Height	1	2	3	4	5
20. Level of physical fitness	1	2	3	4	5
21. Energy level	1	2	3	4	5
22. Overall, how satisfied are you with the way you look?					

Men and women also differ significantly in their responses to the body parts questionnaire that you completed. In a Melpomene study on body image, we were able to predict the sex of a respondent just by looking at the number of positive responses to the assessment of these body parts. Men frequently chose the most positive response, "I consider myself fortunate," while women were rarely more positive than "I am satisfied." How do your responses compare? You may also wish to use this questionnaire with a male friend to verify our results for yourself.

In the Melpomene study, women were more likely to say that body parts not associated with shape were the body parts they like best (i.e., eyes, hair, and overall facial attractiveness). The body parts liked least were thighs (53 percent of the respondents), abdomen (34 percent), and hips (33 percent). Since these are physically active women, perhaps it is not surprising that calves were ranked as a body part liked best by 45 percent of the respondents.

THE STRUGGLE TO "IMPROVE"

Now that you've discovered what most affects your body image, let's take a look at ways we try to "improve" those areas. Whether you try to improve by using makeup, having cosmetic surgery, or losing weight, it's important for you to know *why* you are doing it and to question whether it is the best thing for you.

Makeup

Do most women really spend time worrying about how certain pieces of their bodies look? If we don't, says our society, perhaps we should. Think about a typical hour of network TV. You may see 12 commercials that urge you to fix what's "wrong" with you by using products such as hair coloring, facial cosmetics, hair removers, dry-skin lotion, control-top pantyhose, artificial nails, colored contact lenses, and breath fresheners. Advertisers imply that if we simply "work on" one piece of ourselves at a time, we will realize all our dreams for love and success.

The campaign waged by the cosmetics industry reaches girls at an early age. From their teenage years on, women are encouraged to spend large sums of money on their faces. The illusion is that skillfully applied makeup can hide or eliminate your imperfections so that you are more attractive and desirable. Consider Sandra. She spends a minimum of 45 minutes each morning decorating her face. When she is finished she is pleased with the results and feels much more confident to begin her day as a lawyer. "It makes a big difference professionally if I look well," she says. Jacki, on the other hand, spends a brief 5 minutes giving her face only minimal attention. She says that her competency is more important than her looks.

Both may be right. Jacki's self-confidence in her natural looks, however, saves her more than an hour each day. She says she prefers to spend that time reading or exercising.

Cosmetic Surgery

Most women, as they age, learn to accept those physical features that are not related to weight. Some, however, continue to focus their dissatisfaction on a long nose, sagging eyes, or small breasts. Each year more women consider cosmetic surgery as a way to "improve" the parts they like least. Their desire seems linked to a notion we are all led to believe: that beauty is only a matter of effort, and that perfection is possible if only we can find the means to achieve it.

Have you ever personally wondered about changing a body part through surgery? The variety of women seriously considering it may surprise you. Within the past 15 years we've noticed that women are talking more openly about this option.

In some cases, cosmetic surgery can make a positive difference. Someone who has been truly unhappy with her nose may find that she is happier and more confident as well as more attractive following surgery. Jane, for example, had been uncomfortable with her nose for as long as she could remember. Some newspaper ads plus an article in a magazine convinced her to explore the possibility of surgery in more detail. While she was somewhat embarrassed to be thinking about something that seemed so "vain," she still wanted to know the facts so she could make a wise choice. Not only did she interview several physicians and check out the details of cost and probable outcome, but she also talked with several women who had undergone the same procedure. After a year of asking questions and weighing outcomes, Jane finally scheduled her operation. She reports that the change was just what she had hoped, and that her self-confidence has blossomed as a result.

Sarah's story is quite different. Her husband and friends scoffed when she talked about wanting a face-lift. "You look young and wonderful as you are," they told her. But Sarah was determined and had high expectations for her surgery. "The surgical team was honest in telling me that in my case the improvements would be minimal," Sarah admitted later, "but I still wanted to try it." Unfortunately, Sarah had surgical complications. A new, crooked smile was only one of the negative results which made Sarah angry that she had ever decided to try to "become younger."

Why do women consider cosmetic surgery? Some people believe that the desire to change your appearance must be rooted in deep psychological problems. However, psychologists Judith Burk, Seymour Zelen, and Edward Terino, associated with the California School of Professional Psychology, believe it may be more straightforward than that. According to their tests, they describe the typical surgery candidate as a woman who is "average in terms of general self-esteem, but whose physical self-esteem is lower than average and who seeks the practical solution of cosmetic surgery because of inconsistencies in her self-concept."

Basically, they suggest that a woman has surgery because she has one body part that she likes less than others. Cosmetic surgery is just one of three possible ways she might deal with her dissatisfaction: She can begin to see the body part as less important, she can continue to let it bother her but not do anything, or she can schedule surgery. In their experience, they have seen "stable improvement in esteem of the body as well as the operated body part over time following surgery."

Cosmetic surgery has also been the answer for many women who want some form of breast reconstruction after breast cancer operations. It took Maggie 4 years to decide to have breast reconstruction. Her physicians recommended she wait 2 years following her mastectomy to be sure there were no additional lumps. During that time she became increasingly uncomfortable with her prosthesis: "I was often in a swimsuit, and prostheses were really a bother."

When first exploring the possibility of surgery, she asked for recommendations from two of her friends in a mastectomy support group. She then arranged a session in which she and her husband were able to ask questions of one of the physicians and his team. Maggie felt the team presented excellent information, but she also called back the next day to get some additional questions answered. Because she felt very comfortable with her decision, the time lapse between this visit and the surgery was only 6 weeks.

The first surgery in the two-step process took 2 hours, and Maggie was in the hospital less than 2 days. Her pain was minimal, and she felt well on her way to complete recovery in 1 week. She completed her final surgery as an outpatient 4 months later. Maggie reported that her major complaint was being tired, but that recovery seemed very easy.

She is extremely pleased with the results. "It feels as if I have a breast again!" She thinks that the time between her mastectomy and the decision to have surgery was critical for her. She doesn't think all women should have this surgery, but she has become an advocate due to her positive experience.

Not all implant procedures and recovery go as smoothly as Maggie's. Susan had a mastectomy with tissue reconstruction shortly after her mastectomy. Susan agreed to reconstruction because she wanted to please her husband, whom she knew put great importance on breasts. She allowed herself to be persuaded even though she was not totally comfortable with the decision.

Susan had complications following surgery. Massive infections developed which required additional surgery to remove the infected tissue. Susan's experience points out the importance of researching the pros and cons of cosmetic surgery. Women need to be clear when making decisions about reconstruction. You'll need to be willing to take responsibility for those decisions even when they aren't the same as those of friends, partners, or parents.

Linda Brown Harris, author of *Breast Cancer: A Handbook*, has several reminders for women considering reconstructive surgery:

- Reconstruction cannot duplicate what nature has provided.
- "Simple" or "common" does not necessarily mean without complications. There are no guarantees.
- Exploration of self-esteem, self-acceptance of your body as-is, and self-love are all important in the decision-making process.

While some of us may never consider cosmetic surgery, most of us will continue to try to "improve" our physical appearance in other ways. Sometimes we don't consciously realize what it is about ourselves that we consider most important. Take a few seconds to try a simple but revealing exercise. The directions are easy: Describe yourself.

Describe Yourself

_____

_____

_____

_____

_____

_____

Karen Larkin: Be Happy Now

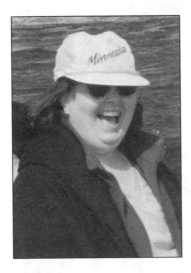

A few weeks ago **Karen Larkin** finished a workout at the Y and was walking to cool down, when a little boy bounded up and said, "Guess what! You're really big. You're even bigger than my mom!" The boy's mortified mother rushed over, apologizing to Karen and scolding the boy severely. Karen smiled and said, "I don't think you heard what I told him. I said, 'Thank you!' He wasn't making a judgment, only an observation." The boy's mother looked surprised and then puzzled. "Wow," she said. "Maybe I should learn to think that way."

Does Karen really feel complimented when someone makes an exclamation about her size? No, she's concerned that her weight may cause legitimate health repercussions, and she'd like to be able to move more freely. Should a child be chastised for making an obvious comment while trying to be friendly? Of course not! Karen thinks that a more open dialogue about size, prejudice, and shame might give way to support and confidence.

Karen spent 2 decades moving from one program to another, trying to "improve" herself. She has lost track of how many hundreds of pounds she has lost and gained. She has spent enough money on weight-loss schemes to have financed a Master's degree. Her self-esteem has been on one long roller-coaster ride. "I've come to believe that in my case acceptance is more appropriate than change," Karen says. "I've started thinking about ways to add to my life instead of taking away. As I shifted my viewpoint, an amazing thing happened: Change occurred. No, I didn't become thin, but I did start claiming my happiness now, as opposed to 'someday, when I'm thinner.'"

Karen has started taking more risks and celebrating her successes. She has learned to nurse her wounds without feeling defeated when things don't go well. She sees now that chocolate-chip cookies and asparagus are both good things. She discovered that exercise sessions are a wonderful chance to daydream. She makes friends easier now.

She has a great job, a comfortable home, and she hopes to become a mom.

Will Karen ever lose weight again? Maybe. But if she does, the challenge will be about just that—weight. It's no longer about self-worth. Right now she does not believe a safe, effective treatment for obesity exists. But research continues, and she has learned to never say never. In the meantime, she reduces the risk factors that she can control, taking things easier and remembering to laugh. Will her own child ever say anything in public that embarrasses her? She hopes so!

If you are like the majority of white women, you answered with physical attributes rather than character descriptions. You mentioned features that you feel are distinctive, or even central to who you are. Regardless of other personal descriptors, you probably also mentioned weight. A recent study in *Essence* magazine suggests weight is also becoming an issue for more black women.

A Weighty Issue

The serious impact that weight has on many women's lives is highlighted in a 1984 survey by *Glamour* magazine. Women were asked which they would prefer: (1) a date with a man they admire, (2) seeing an old friend, (3) a promotion or success at work, or (4) losing weight. The greatest percentage chose losing weight. In a 1987 *Ms.* magazine survey, losing weight was not a number one priority, but 64.4 percent agreed with the statement "I would like myself better if I were thinner." Obviously, weight and body shape, or rather, a woman's perception of her shape, are critical to how she feels about herself as a person. While there is no study to back up our belief that there has been a subtle change since that time, we're encouraged by a 1993 *Glamour* article titled "Your Weight, Your Health" which advises: Take control now. Trade the ups and downs of dieting for a focus on weight maintenance.

What weight should you try to maintain? How do you decide what is a desirable weight for you? Many women see themselves as overweight and undesirable when they are actually within the "desirable weight range" for their age. But who decides what is a desirable or ideal weight? Quantitative data on weight, both actual and ideal, first appeared around the turn of the century. The first table compiled in

1912 by an insurance company became known as the Metropolitan Desirable Weight Table. It set standards of height and weight by bone structure using the groups with the lowest death rates as the ideal. This table, which was updated and revised in 1931, 1943, 1959, and 1983, has become the standard most doctors and the general public usually choose to determine relative fatness or thinness. Although this standard is open to question, millions of Americans rely on it to see how they measure up.

A more recent chart has been provided by the U.S. Department of Agriculture (USDA). Its 1991 Dietary Guidelines for Americans "Acceptable Weights for Men and Women" was adapted from the 1959 Metropolitan Desirable Weight Table and lists weights that increase at every height after age 35 (see right side of chart on p. 59). This table does not differentiate by sex, but rather suggests, for example, that both men and women who are 5 feet, 4 inches, weigh an "acceptable amount" between 111 and 146 pounds. After age 35, an acceptable weight range for the same height is 122 to 157 pounds.

Dr. Reubin Andres, clinical director of the Gerontology Research Center of the National Institute on Aging, contends that the Metropolitan Life charts are "too high for young people, too low for middle aged and older, and just right for those in their early forties." Gerontology experts tell us that it is reasonable for our weight to increase as we age. Most of us will not fit into our wedding dress 25 years later. One Melpomene Institute volunteer said that she had only recently given away clothes she had worn when she was 47 and several pounds lighter; now 53 and still very trim and athletic, Miriam has finally become comfortable with her new weight and decided that the clothes will never again fit. Unfortunately, many women are not as accepting of their normal shifts in body weight that come with aging.

Weight alone is not as good an index of your healthy weight as determining your body mass index (BMI). This is done by dividing a person's weight in kilograms by her height in meters squared. Therefore, a woman 5 feet, 4 inches, weighing 145 pounds has a BMI of 25%. This is still in the healthy range. The chart on page 60 lists BMIs for various weights and heights.

BODY FAT MEASUREMENTS: MOTIVATOR OR MILLSTONE?

Many of us judge what we should or shouldn't eat by the most current reading on the scale. When taken to the extreme, weight scales can

How Weight Guidelines Changed

Desirable body weight ranges issued by the United States Departments of Agriculture and Health and Human Services. In 1990 men and women were grouped together and broken down by age, suggesting that it is desirable for women over 35 to gain weight. Heights are without shoes; weights are without clothes.

	1985			1990	
Height	Men	Women	Height	19 to 34	35 and over
4'10"		92-121			
4'11"		95-124			
5'0"		98-127	5'0"	97-128	108-138
5'1"	105-134	101-130	5'1"	101-132	111-143
5'2"	108-137	104-134	5'2"	104-137	115-148
5'3"	111-141	107-138	5'3"	107-141	119-152
5'4"	114-145	110-142	5'4"	111-146	122-157
5'5"	117-149	114-146	5'5"	114-150	126-162
5'6"	121-154	118-150	5'6"	118-155	130-167
5'7"	125-159	122-154	5'7"	121-160	134-172
5'8"	129-163	126-159	5'8"	125-164	138-178
5'9"	133-167	130-164	5'9"	129-169	142-183
5'10"	137-172	134-169	5'10"	132-174	146-188
5'11"	141-177		5'11"	136-179	151-194
6'0"	145-182		6'0"	140-184	155-199
6'1"	149-187		6'1"	144-189	159-205
6'2"	153-192		6'2"	148-195	164-210
6'3"	157-197		6'3"	152-200	168-216
			6'4"	156-205	173-222
			6'5"	160-211	177-228
			6'6"	164-216	182-234

How to Gauge Your Healthy Weight

Body Mass Index Height (inches)	19	20	21	22	23	24	25	26	27	28	29	30	35	40
						Body weight (pounds)								
58	91	96	100	105	110	115	119	124	129	134	138	143	167	191
59	94	99	104	109	114	119	124	128	133	138	143	148	173	198
60	97	102	107	112	118	123	128	133	138	143	148	153	179	204
61	100	106	111	116	122	127	132	137	143	148	153	158	185	211
62	104	109	115	120	126	131	136	142	147	153	158	164	191	218
63	107	113	118	124	130	135	141	146	152	158	163	169	197	225
64	110	116	122	128	134	140	145	151	157	163	169	174	204	232
65	114	120	126	132	138	144	150	156	162	168	174	180	210	240
66	118	124	130	136	142	148	155	161	167	173	179	186	216	247
67	121	127	134	140	146	153	159	166	172	178	185	191	223	255
68	125	131	138	144	151	158	164	171	177	184	190	197	230	262
69	128	135	142	149	155	162	169	176	182	189	196	203	236	270
70	132	139	146	153	160	167	174	181	188	195	202	207	243	278
71	136	143	150	157	165	172	179	186	193	200	208	215	250	286
72	140	147	154	162	169	177	184	191	199	206	213	221	258	294

become instruments of torture. A method that may more accurately document your fitness level is to measure your body fat. The summary of methods of measuring body fat that follows in this section can help you decide if it is useful for you. Avoid it if you suspect one more tyrannical number will keep you from having a good, healthy body image.

What are body fat measurements? Is it possible to get such a reading at an annual medical checkup? Can you do it yourself? What methods are available, and how accurate are they?

Underwater Weighing

Some researchers still consider underwater weighing to be the most accurate method to measure body fat. Before taking the measurement, a technician uses a special apparatus to measure your residual oxygen—that is, the oxygen left after you expel all the air from your lungs. You are then lowered into a tank of water on a chair attached to a scale. After recording your underwater weight, the technician raises you from the water and then repeats the procedure about six times to assure accurate measurement. One problem is that because people's bone mineral content and body water varies, this method leads to an overestimation of body fat in older women and an underestimation in an athletic population. The method is also somewhat tedious and requires sophisticated equipment and skilled technicians.

Skin Fold

Research has also validated the usefulness of skin fold measurement to determine body fat. In this method, the technician uses calipers to measure the thickness of pinched skin at specified points on your body. Generalized equations for predicting body density were developed by researchers Jackson and Pollock and described in the *British Journal of Nutrition* in 1978. These equations have become accepted and are widely used by the Y's and other fitness centers.

Computer Testing

In the mid-eighties, a third method of measuring body fat became available. This method is based on how much fluid your cells contain

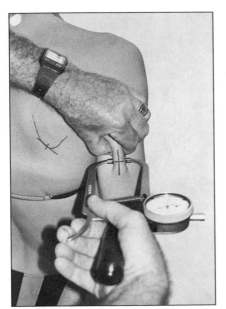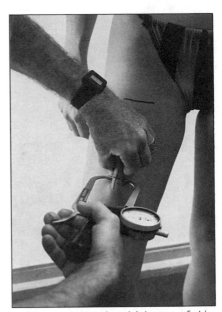

In skin fold measurement, calipers are used to measure the thickness of skin pinched at certain points of the body, such as the arm or thigh.

and how quickly an electrical charge can move through them. Electricity moves fastest through fat-free cells because they are primarily made up of fluid, whereas fat cells have only 14 percent of this conducting medium. To take the measurement, a technician hooks electrodes up to your body and introduces a low-voltage charge. As the charge travels through your body, it is slowed down by the fat compartments but moves freely through the fat-free cells. By analyzing how easily the charge passes through your cells, the device can estimate how much of your body is made up of fat.

This method relies on accurate knowledge or measurement of body weight, height, and age—all factors in the formula used to derive the percentage of body fat. The success of this method, as with the other two described, depends on how careful and experienced the operator is. In addition, it is not accurate for a heavy woman or for the competitive athlete. Also, because fluid is so important in the test, dehydration can cause errors.

Which Method Is Best?

With all the possibilities for error, is it worth trying to get your body fat measured? What is the best method? Melpomene Institute has conducted research using both underwater weighing and skin fold measurements. Our findings suggest that accurate caliper measurement can be effectively used in the research setting. We've also seen evidence that as long as health professionals and physical educators are adequately trained, they can take accurate skin fold readings at hospitals and health clubs. Since it is also considerably faster and more economical than underwater weighing, skin fold measurement is our method of choice. We urge you to be wary, however, of the inexpensive calipers advertised in fitness magazines. Most are not useful at all; they are poorly calibrated, and, since some practice is needed for accuracy, it is difficult to perform the test on yourself or friends. Your best bet is to be measured by a professional. And, if you want to recheck your measurements at a later date, try to have it done by the same person or at the same facility.

A warning here: If you are like many women who experience a 2- to 5-pound water-weight gain just before their periods, your body fat percentage may also be influenced by the stage of your menstrual cycle. Diane Wakat, PhD, professor and nutritional counselor at the University of Virginia, finds that specific site measurements might vary by as much as 3mm on certain days, resulting in a body fat that fluctuates 3-5 percent. According to Wakat, most women can expect their body fat to be highest during the 4-6 days before their periods. Coaches who set specific body fat limits for their athletes (e.g., below 18 percent) don't always recognize the fact that a woman may measure 18 percent one week and 23 percent the next. The water weight that causes the fluctuation will also affect girth measurements and computerized methods of determining body fat.

Well, you may be thinking, it sounds as if all methods have margins of error; it doesn't seem as if any of these readings are absolute. Why not just continue to evaluate myself by how much I weigh? What if I discover that my body fat percentage is "worse" than my weight?

Even though the measurement of body fat has some problems, it is a better way to measure fitness than scale weight is. Weight as measured on a scale says little about the composition of that weight. Since muscle weighs more than fat, a muscular person will weigh more on a scale. A well-toned, muscled body, however, looks better and burns calories more efficiently than a flabby body. Look at yourself in the mirror. The way you look depends in large part on your fitness. It always surprises women to learn that someone who weighs 145 pounds can have only 19 percent body fat. On the other hand, sedentary women who believed they were a good weight may find their body fat to be higher than they would like it to be.

The problem is that we have all been socialized to have some idea of what "fat" is on a scale and so are apt to judge our own body image on that basis. Body fat percentages are new to us, and we don't yet know what a "good" body fat percentage would be for our age, height, and weight. To help you key in on this, you'll need some idea of the range of body fats in both active and sedentary populations.

Putting Body Fat Percentages in Perspective

To avoid letting body fat measurements become another unreachable goal, it's important for you to know that "normal" body fat for nonathletic women is 28-30 percent. A figure of 22-25 percent represents fitness and relative slimness. Covert Bailey, who published a newsletter on body fat issues, states that: "Adult women below 22 percent body fat are rare. I see plenty of them because our program attracts healthy athletic people, but they represent a small fraction of the population. There are only a few body fat studies on very young children, but the evidence is that pre-puberty girls (who) are normally active stay below 15 percent body fat. After puberty, female fat levels tend to rise, and rise, and rise, stopping at a healthy 22 percent only for those who exercise regularly."

Bailey, who has measured the body fat of many athletic women using the underwater weighing method, finds that a woman needs to be "professionally involved" with exercise to achieve the 18 percent level desired by many. Aerobic dance instructors and women who regularly compete as runners or triathletes are more likely to achieve these levels, he says, but even they usually modify their diets to maintain the weight.

Unfortunately, Bailey's information is not common knowledge. In our research with physically active women, we are finding that women would prefer to have a somewhat lower percentage of body fat than what is considered average. This was highlighted by a Melpomene study conducted with low-mileage runners who on average said they wanted to measure 19 percent body fat. Even more damaging was the fact that many of these women were comparing themselves with the few, elite distance runners they had read about who average 13 percent body fat. As long as they were exercising, the women felt that they should be able to "achieve" a 15 percent or lower body fat reading, which is unrealistic and probably unhealthy for most.

When the Melpomene staff measured body fat at a women's YWCA race in 1985, we heard firsthand how important these measurements were becoming to women. Their conversations with one another underscored the need for better education about body fat. "Body fat is a better measure of fitness," said one, "so I plan to put more importance on this reading than on my scale weight." Said another, "I'm hoping that my body fat measurement will finally tell me I'm not overweight, or at least not overfat. If my body fat reading is 20 percent then I can stop worrying."

How do you react to these statements? At Melpomene we're concerned. Too many women spend their lives searching for an outside, objective source that will tell them that their bodies are OK. As long as their internal self-confidence and body image remains low, we believe that even a "good" reading won't stop the search. In many cases, physically active women know they look and feel better because of their activity, and yet they still worry. Using body fat numbers as evidence that you are not meeting some false, external standard can be self-defeating.

Kay, laughingly but with some embarrassment, shared the fact that after a year of exercise she had become much happier with her body. "I had lost very little weight on the scale," she said, "but my clothes fit differently. One of my sons said he really liked the muscles on my legs. I felt pretty good and thought that I would verify the changes with a body fat measurement. The club measured me at 28 percent! Since I had just been reading my first runner's magazine about women who were 13 percent body fat, I was really discouraged. To be honest, I went out and bought a fad diet book. I've been following that diet for 3 weeks now, and the only results I see are that I'm crabbier and harder to live with, and my running is worse. I don't have the energy."

If you choose to measure your weight or body fat, consider measuring yourself only one time a year. Ninety-nine percent of respondents to a 1993 Melpomene/*Self* magazine study of women aged 40-66 said they knew what had happened to their weight in the past year, yet 24 percent seldom weighed themselves, and an additional 25 percent weighed only a couple of times a month. Since most of us can tell what is happening to our weight by the way our clothes look, why worry about what some number says from one day to the next?

Keep in mind that the healthy range for body fat may be far broader than either the media or the medical profession would have us believe. Many experts agree with Kelly Brownell, a Yale University psychology professor who has written extensively about dieting and size, that the best weight for most people is the lowest they've been able to maintain for a year as an adult without struggling.

Yet a study published in the *Journal of the American Medical Association* in 1995 once again complicated the picture. Authors Walter Willett, JoAnn Manson, Meir Stampfer, and colleagues concluded that higher levels of body weight within the "normal" range, as well as modest weight gains after 18 years of age, appear to increase risks of coronary heart disease in middle-aged women. Headlines across the country sounded the alarm. "At Midlife, Added Pounds Mean Added Risk"; "Women's Weight Gain Points to Coronary Risk." We are skeptical of the real meaning of the statistics and disturbed by their impact. Many women called Melpomene in the weeks following the article's publication. One woman said: "After years of dieting, I had just accepted the fact that 130 pounds is a weight that I can maintain. I'm 49 and I know the weights suggested, 110 pounds for my 5-foot, 2-inch frame, are unrealistic. Yet, this new information makes me worried I'll die of a heart attack." She was worried her weight might not be just a body image issue but a health issue.

DIETING: THE NATIONAL PASTIME

Living up to the standards of "desirable weight" can be a lifelong struggle for many women. Although figures vary according to the study or survey quoted, somewhere between 40 and 50 percent of American women are on a diet of some sort at any given time. The diet industry brings in $33 billion a year. Some of these women are convinced that 180, 200, or 240 pounds is not a healthy weight. But many women who diet weigh 105, 120, or 140 pounds. Most of them are dieting because they think they will look better.

Wayne Calloway, MD, an obesity specialist at the Mayo clinic, has spoken about the healthy obese. He suggests that chronic unhappiness associated with repeated attempts at weight control may shorten your life. And there is little reason to believe that preoccupation with weight diminishes with age. In our 1993 Melpomene/*Self* magazine study of menopausal women, those respondents who considered themselves underweight were more likely to believe their feelings of happiness were better or much better than other women their age. Additionally, women who had lost weight during the previous year were more likely to say their happiness was "much better." It is frequently this preoccupation, rather than a therapeutic need to lose weight, that encourages dieting behavior. Melpomene studies indicate that women who diet are far less satisfied with their bodies than those who do not.

How often do you diet? If you are among those women who can say "never," you will want to read this section to gain a better understanding of friends who are always dieting. If, on the other hand, you sometimes or frequently diet, this section may help you evaluate whether or not you really need to diet and what you should expect.

When you decide you "need to diet" are you talking about a formal plan or something as simple as restricting snacks? Look at the following choices and identify the methods you would choose to reduce weight.

Popular Ways of Reducing Weight (not all recommended)

- Decrease size of portions
- Eliminate carbohydrates
- Avoid sweets
- Count calories
- Reduce fat intake
- Eliminate snacks
- Increase physical activity
- Try a popular diet
- Purge
- Enroll in a weight reduction program
- Fast
- Increase caffeine intake
- Start to smoke, or increase number of cigarettes smoked

The Problem With Weight Reduction Diets

Is there a good weight reduction diet? Some of the choices listed above are obviously more healthy than others, yet all are methods currently used by American women. What is the long-term success rate of dieting? Kelly Brownell says, "If one defines successful treatment as return to ideal body weight and maintenance for five years, a person is more likely to recover from almost any form of cancer than from obesity."

Available research shows that people may lose weight while participating in a program, but many individuals regain one-third to two-thirds of intentionally lost weight within one year and regain the rest of the weight within 5 years.

Rather than talking about dieting for weight loss as a short-term fix, we need to talk about making a lifelong commitment to healthy eating that will contribute to weight management. When you consider losing weight, you need to consider the possible health benefits of a lower body weight, the difficulty of the task, and the potential harmful physical and psychological effects of weight loss programs.

Nutritionist Joan Vogel warns against diets that include one or all of the following tricks for quick weight loss:

- Eating fewer carbohydrates while consuming large amounts of fats and protein
- Eating only special foods and/or food supplements
- Drastically reducing the number of calories you consume

One of the main reasons these strategies tend to fail is that they concentrate on what you shouldn't eat instead of recommending eating habits that are healthy. Denying yourself certain foods is a quick fix rather than a new lifestyle. Until you develop eating habits with which you can comfortably live for a lifetime, claims Vogel, any weight loss will be a temporary one. Besides being just plain ineffective, some of these diets can also wreak havoc on your body.

When you are on a low-carbohydrate diet, your body will be burning fats for fuel. Since fats are not efficient producers of energy, waste products in the form of ketones are produced. This influx of ketones causes your kidneys to excrete more water and body fluids, while the rest of your body experiences a feeling of fatigue. Because you are eating fewer carbohydrates, chances are you are filling in with higher percentages of fats and proteins. The connection between high-fat foods and higher blood cholesterol has been well documented and publicized. What you may not have heard about is that high-fat, low–protein diets can also leave your body hungry for calcium and minerals such as iron. Vogel warns: "The most destructive aspect of decreased protein is the breakdown of the body's muscle tissue to satisfy energy requirements. During this process, some of the body fat is lost but lean tissue or lean body mass is also reduced, causing a loss of strength."

The most extreme starvation diets are self-limiting. Usually the dieter quits because the side effects of fatigue, irritability, mood swings, and depression become unmanageable. One of the most devastating consequences of low-calorie diets is that they eventually reduce your resting metabolic rate, making it more difficult for you to burn off excess calories and lose weight.

This lowered metabolic rate is a consequence of all diets. To keep you from losing too much weight, your body begins to burn fuel more slowly, stretching every serving you give it. Thanks to your new metabolic rate (15 to 30 percent lower than normal), you don't need to spend as many calories to accomplish a given amount of work. Naturally, and by design, this added efficiency makes it harder for you to lose pounds.

The same law of diminishing returns applies to physical exercise and weight loss. By the second or third year of regular exercise, most women find that their bodies become accustomed to the extra energy drain. The body again becomes more efficient. Those who say they have to eat less or exercise more to maintain a desired weight are often reporting the truth!

Disordered Eating

Food and the struggle to control eating play a major role in the lives of many women. Consider Susan and Sally, who struck up a conversation at their children's tennis meet. "Well, I finally did it," exclaimed Sally, "I signed up for Weight Watchers!" Susan, who didn't know Sally well, was somewhat incredulous; Sally was a thin, attractive woman who did not look as if she needed to lose weight. As they talked further, Sally revealed that she weighed herself two or three times every day, and spent at least an hour a day worrying about food. A pound or 2 was cause for concern, 3 or 4 pounds meant that she canceled plans to meet a friend for lunch. Although she always made up other excuses, the real reason for her change in plans was that she "felt too fat." Unfortunately, eating to fulfill hunger or for pleasure is not a key element in many women's lives.

Being an athlete can further complicate attitudes toward food and fat. A woman who perceives herself primarily as an athlete may link her self-worth to sports performance. She may feel that she has much to lose if she should gain weight and be unable to do well in her sport. She constantly faces the internal threat: "If I become fat, I will not be an athlete any longer, and if I am not an athlete, then who am I?" Young women who have been in competitive athletics for many years may find the thought of not competing especially frightening, thus reinforcing their struggle to stay thin. One college athlete tells of her experience as a member of a women's crew team:

> My first year rowing I had a healthy experience. My coach always told us we looked great, and the emphasis was on being strong and healthy instead of thin. That year I gained weight and felt better about myself than I ever had. I was the strongest I had ever been, and I was in the best shape of my life. It was a real confidence-builder.
>
> The following summer I joined a boat club in order to stay in shape until fall. The coach there was used to coaching lightweight rowers. Instead of tailoring her coaching style to accommodate us, she pressured us to lose weight. At first I took it as a challenge—I could lose that 5 pounds and make weight, so I did it. Then she pressured me to lose more. I joined a few other women who were going on sweat runs and not eating after practice. The

only thing that seemed to matter was making sure we all averaged 125 pounds or less in order to make weight. I completely lost perspective and put my health and safety at risk. I became obsessed about calories and became thin and unhappy. I also lost my self-confidence. None of us were effective rowers—our bodies were too tired. When I went back to school in the fall, my coach told me I had to gain some weight, and I was more than happy to oblige.

From Disordered Eating to Eating Disorders

Happily, this athlete received good advice from her college coach. She also realized the negative aspects of severe weight control. With the support of the coach, friends, and family she avoided developing a true eating disorder. Some are not as lucky. Some high school and collegiate athletes feel they have little control over their lives, and that parents, coaches, and teachers are at the helm instead. Chances are they may be striving to do well at all things in order to please the other people in their lives. Not eating is a subtle way of exerting control over both oneself and others, and may be chosen when the athlete sees no alternative.

How does a preoccupation with weight or a problem with food cross the line and become an eating disorder? Experts are unsure but agree that an eating disorder is more than just dieting that has gotten out of control. For women with eating disorders, the drive to be thin becomes the focal point of their identity, sometimes to the exclusion of all else.

It is important to distinguish between the eating disorders of anorexia nervosa and bulimia. Anorexia is the denial of food to the point of near starvation and resulting weight loss. The anorexic has a distorted body image, often seeing herself as fat even though her weight loss has left her looking emaciated. She typically lives with an intense fear of becoming fat. While it may seem that the anorexic is not interested in food, the opposite is actually true. She may have an incredible amount of nutritional knowledge which she uses to avoid unnecessary fat or calories in her diet. She may also prepare elaborate meals for others or offer gifts of food but will not eat the treats herself. The typical anorexic is a high achiever from a good family, who is obedient, over-motivated, and successful academically. Anorexia seems to be a way for the compliant person to react against pressures to be perfect.

Bulimia is an eating disorder that involves episodes of binge eating of high-calorie foods. A person on a binge will consume anywhere from 2,000 to 20,000 calories at a time. Afterwards, the bulimic is overcome with guilt and attempts to negate the food she has eaten by purging it. Purging may take the form of vomiting, fasting, use of laxatives or diuretics, or even excessive exercise.

Bulimia is more common than anorexia, and some anorexics may become bulimic over time. Since many women hide their eating disorders, it's hard to document the extent of the problem. Molly O'Neill, in a January 1991 *New York Times* article, reports that 15 percent of all college women struggle with eating disorders.

Many psychological and social issues surround eating disorders, including self-esteem and family expectations. Women who are athletic face additional issues and pressures that may contribute to an eating disorder. For example, women who compete in sports such as running, dance, or gymnastics may believe that they would look better or perform better if they weighed less. Participants in these "thin-body" sports often find themselves involved in unhealthy weight loss practices; eventually, some of these women may develop an eating disorder.

A unique aspect of exercise in relation to eating disorders is that physical activity may be used as a purge. It is not unusual for the woman with an eating disorder to engage in excessive exercise in an attempt to negate food that has been eaten or will be eaten in the future. This purge component of exercise raises interesting questions as we learn more about body image and eating disorders. It is often difficult to tell whether an athlete exercises to become thin or to stay thin, or if that athlete is thin in order to be good at her sport. Even after making that distinction, we still don't know at what point exercise becomes excessive, or when it can be considered part of an eating disorder or purging. These questions are often difficult for coaches or health-care providers working with athletes to answer.

In large part because of the increased media coverage describing the dangers of eating disorders, many coaches say they are more careful when talking to their athletes about weight loss. Coaches are in a unique position to influence young athletes, both as role models and as sources of guidance. A coach's insensitive comments can be damaging, especially if they play into the doubts and misperceptions that many athletes have about their bodies. One athlete told us: "At age 14, my cycling coach told me I was 'fat' in front of my entire team . . . At 5 feet, 5 inches, 124 pounds, I was

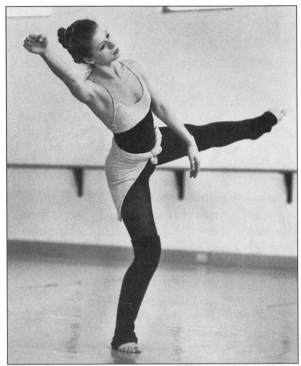

© Courtesy of the *Daily Illini*

How thin is too thin? Coaches and teachers need to be aware of potential problems with women who participate in "thin-body" sports or activities.

not fat, but my self-esteem was so low that I simply believed him. After all, he was the coach." Comments like this one often incite a round of weight-loss attempts that may someday develop into an eating disorder. Being aware of this possibility is essential for anyone who works with active young women. These days, we are inundated with requests from coaches, trainers, and athletes for information about better nutrition, not weight loss. Instead of urging their athletes to eat less, coaches wisely try to focus on eating smarter.

In 1987 the NCAA decided to play a leadership role in providing information to coaches and athletes. In conjunction with the United States Olympic Committee they developed and distributed a program called "Nutrition and Eating Disorders in College Athletics." In 1990 three video programs were also produced and distributed to athletic directors at the collegiate level that address the issue of eating disorders and offer specific suggestions for both coaches and athletes. The fact that the problem is recognized and discussed is a positive step forward.

It is important to emphasize that disordered eating and eating disorders are not unique to physically active women. At Melpomene we have been dismayed when newspaper articles suggest that becoming an athlete is dangerous. Indeed, eating disorders among the nonathletic population often go unrecognized and untreated far longer.

It seems to us that more research is needed to understand the true size and scope of the issue as well as how to treat it best. One of the problems is in identifying women with distorted eating patterns. A bulimic, for instance, often hides her eating habits, making it hard to offer her help at the early stages. Once the problem surfaces, friends and family are often poorly equipped to help her find treatment. Thankfully, because of the publicity about eating disorders in the last few years, more seminars and books are now available on how to identify and help eating-disordered women. National organizations that provide this sort of information are listed in the bibliography. If you are concerned about your own eating habits or those of a friend or daughter, it's time to gather information and make some changes.

ABANDON THE DIET MENTALITY: THINK HEALTHY LIVING INSTEAD

Both healthy eating and exercise play a role in keeping us healthy and fit. We've included here some practical tips to help you do both well.

Eating Healthy

Although there are hundreds of books and articles on eating and dieting, most of us do not have accurate information about food choices. Studies that measure how much we actually know about calorie content in foods, for instance, suggest that our estimates are frequently inaccurate. Sonia Blackman, Timothy Mertz, and Robert Singer, associates with the Center for Social and Behavioral Science Research at the University of California, asked 53 men and 82 women whose average age was 24 to estimate calories in various foods. Most people were accurate when estimating the number of calories in main meals but were way off base when it came to desserts and snacks. They were much more likely to think that desserts were more caloric than main entrees.

The best idea is to forget calories and instead think about healthy eating. The four food groups many of us remember as kids have been reformatted as the food guide pyramid shown below. Six food groups appear in the pyramid because each group provides some but not all of the essential nutrients. A healthy diet includes foods from all of the groups. It's particularly important to eat five or more servings of fruits and vegetables each day. A low intake of fruits and vegetables is directly associated with an increased risk of chronic diseases, particularly cancer.

However, "Eating in America Today, a Dietary Pattern and Intake Report," issued in 1994, indicates that for most Americans the "tumbling" pyramid shown on the next page better reflects how we truly eat. The tumbling pyramid is top-heavy due to the large number of servings of fats/oils/sweets, which are greater than any of the servings from the vegetable, fruit, milk, and meat groups.

There are no good or bad foods. Eating to satisfy hunger and enjoyment should enable you to eat healthfully without feeling guilty. Are you likely to skip dessert but have a small second helping of a casserole or salad with dressing? You may be surprised to learn that the dessert you are longing for may have fewer calories than the stroganoff you

The USDA Food Pyramid—How We Ought to Eat

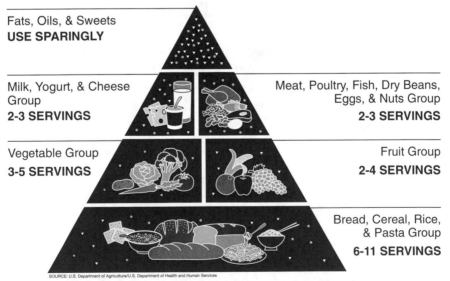

Fats, Oils, & Sweets
USE SPARINGLY

Milk, Yogurt, & Cheese Group
2-3 SERVINGS

Meat, Poultry, Fish, Dry Beans, Eggs, & Nuts Group
2-3 SERVINGS

Vegetable Group
3-5 SERVINGS

Fruit Group
2-4 SERVINGS

Bread, Cereal, Rice, & Pasta Group
6-11 SERVINGS

SOURCE: U.S. Department of Agriculture/U.S. Department of Health and Human Services

From U.S. Department of Agriculture/U. S. Department of Health and Human Services.

The Tumbling Pyramid—How We Do Eat

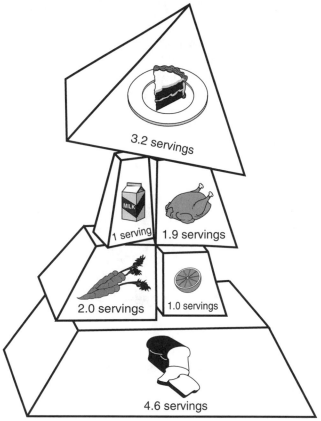

3.2 servings

1 serving   1.9 servings

2.0 servings   1.0 servings

4.6 servings

Adapted from the U.S. Department of Agriculture/National Meat Board.

took instead. If you're one of those people for whom dinner is not complete without dessert, you may be better off eating less of the main course and "saving" some calories for dessert. As Alice, one of our members, says, "It doesn't make any sense for me to totally cut out desserts. I know that I'll end up eating something sweet before I go to bed."

For Alice, enjoying her dessert is a wise decision. Many women probably unnecessarily limit certain foods because they have mentally classified them as "good" or "bad." Changing your own attitudes about food will make you more aware of how many people are overly concerned with food choices.

Ways to Eat Nutritiously

- Keep a variety of foods on hand, so you can choose what you want to eat when you're hungry.
- Add new foods to what you now eat, rather than worrying about what not to eat.
- Take time to enjoy every bite.
- Eat regularly rather than skipping meals or going hungry.
- Go to a farmer's market or produce stand to buy fresh fruits and vegetables.

Reprinted from *Living in a Healthy Body, A New Look at Health and Weight.*

Does Exercise Make a Difference?

Becoming physically active can change your body shape by toning and hardening your muscles and lowering your body fat over time. It may not mean that you weigh less on the scale, however. In fact, since muscle weighs more than fat, some women's weight may increase slightly with exercise. Lyle is a good example. When she started exercising, she was not overweight, but she was overfat. Three weeks after she began running and weight training, she noticed that her clothes fit more loosely around her waist. After 6 weeks, friends and colleagues remarked on her changed body. Expecting to find a major drop in weight, Lyle was dismayed to see that the scale reading had crept up. Exercise had burned the fat, but it built up muscle, causing her scale weight to climb. Fortunately, the positive comments Lyle received convinced her that she was moving in the right direction and did not need to be dismayed by her weight gain.

If you are like most women, you can expect to lose some weight after taking up a regular exercise program. You should probably not expect to lose more than 5 to 15 pounds in a year's time, however. At first this change will occur without major changes to your diet. As you become more skilled or perhaps competitive in your activity, you may want to drop more weight. In our studies, we found that women runners were still concerned with weight, even after they had become wonderfully fit. This desire seems to stem from the notion that being thinner will improve performance. Although this has never been proven conclusively, the anecdotal "evidence" has made it a powerful myth. Women who become competitive quickly learn that if someone says, "You're looking good," they mean that you have lost several pounds.

Once you pass the level of change that occurs naturally with exercise, we suggest you forget about "achieving" some preconceived notion of your ideal weight or body fat percentage. Don't fall into the trap Ellen describes. Ellen, 56, is a good example of someone who exercises regularly, yet still worries excessively about her weight and food intake. Ellen grew up on a farm where physical activity was expected and often required. She ate balanced meals, and though never thin, she remained at a healthy 27 percent body fat until she was 49. While going through menopause, she noticed that she was gaining weight although her diet remained the same. Cutting down on calories didn't seem to help. At the same time, Ellen realized that the stress of her job seemed to be causing headaches and backaches. A friend encouraged her to go walking as part of an informal Saturday morning group. Skeptical at first, Ellen soon found that she loved the exercise and was meeting new women with whom she could share thoughts and concerns. In the first 6 months, she not only had fewer headaches and backaches, but also noticed a difference in how clothes fit and how she looked.

Two years later, Ellen found that her body had learned to use calories more efficiently so that exercise was not enough. She decided she needed to limit calories in order to maintain a body fat that she felt was acceptable. Ellen began to agonize over the calories of everything she ate. After struggling for a year she found an understanding psychologist to help her accept a new, more realistic body weight.

The problem of distorted body image had more severe consequences for Beth. Beth started running in her late twenties. Her goal was twofold: to lose some weight and to become a competent runner. She had several running friends whom she admired for their thin bodies and their strength. Beth achieved her goal of competence in the first 2 years of running. She often placed in her age category in local races and continually improved her times. Initially she also experienced some weight loss as a result of running and changing her diet. But Beth also loved to eat and had certain food desires that she found impossible to curb. She eventually became bulimic, eating vast quantities of cookies, ice cream, and crackers in binges that she hid from her closest friends.

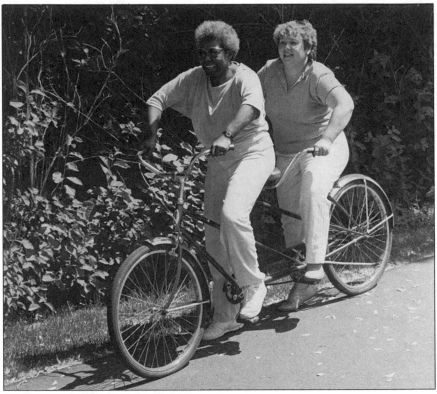

Once your body has adapted naturally to your exercise routine, forget about "achieving" a preconceived notion of your ideal weight—you'll find it's not "ideal," after all.

These reactions, fortunately, are exceptions rather than the rule. For most women, taking up exercise helps them to put less importance on the issue of weight. Women participating in a 1990 Melpomene study indicated that physical activity often improves overall body image and self-esteem. Some women talked about a changed attitude toward calories. For example, "I'm proud to say that my attitudes about myself and food have been shifting; I realize that I paid too much attention to food and calories in the past . . . I really don't think in terms of calories very much anymore. I've become more concerned with good nutrition."

Others have begun to look at their bodies in new ways. Some talked about new perceptions: "I've decided to appreciate my curves and have decided they are womanly rather than fat!" Others emphasized the function of their bodies:

"I feel stronger and more fit. I like looking more muscular instead of flabby."

"I'm active for sanity and vanity—the sense of accomplishment, feeling of well-being, keeping my body in shape."

"I like finding out that my body can do things it couldn't do before."

"Physical activity helps improve my self-esteem and feeling of power and independence."

"I feel very positive; I feel strong and appreciate how my body looks."

"I feel better about my body so I can tackle almost anything."

BODY IMAGE AND SELF-ESTEEM

It may be surprising that the way we feel about our bodies does not always correlate with how we feel about our self-worth or self-esteem. Psychologists have found that we can have a good body image and low self-esteem, or vice versa. Body image is only one of the factors that contribute to self-esteem; there are many others. Sometimes, a good body image is not enough to boost self-esteem above the "threshold of worthiness."

Consider Jane, for example, who had a body that men admired and other women envied. She was always able to eat whatever she wanted and therefore never worried or even thought much about food. Jane grew up in a home where good eating habits were established early; the meals were well balanced, low in fat and protein, and high in complex carbohydrates. When Jane was in junior high school, some of her friends remarked on the lack of junk food in her house; Jane confessed that she envied them and loved to come to their homes to "gorp out." For the most part, however, Jane found no reason to change the way she ate. When many of her friends were becoming heavier and very concerned about body appearance and fat, Jane grew tall and wondered why everyone else spent so much time worrying about food. Her good body, however, did not insulate Jane from other problems. She was not a good student and constantly fought to get good grades. She had difficulty getting along with an older sister who envied Jane's slim-without-a-struggle body. She had few friends and began to blame her good body for her loneliness, even though the issues were clearly more complex. By the end of her first year in college, Jane's outward appearance fooled many people who could not believe that her self-image was so vulnerable.

By the same token, a bad body image will not necessarily drag down a buoyant self-esteem. Consider Kisha, who did not have the perfect body. Even her youngest baby pictures showed someone who was decidedly fat. Some of her earliest memories include being called "Fats" in kindergarten and being chosen last for the teams at recess. It seemed to her that people spent far too much time assessing her body instead of her talents. She could, after all, bat better than most boys, and her sturdy body was often an asset in touch football. Kisha also enjoyed books, photography, and school. She spent a lot of time reading, and for several years had few friends because she was not only fat but also a good student. Kisha learned to downplay grades without ever giving up her love of learning or her drive to succeed. In high school, she discovered she had acting talent and began to develop friends and self-confidence. Thus, even though she dieted constantly and was clearly dissatisfied with her body image, her self-esteem was far better than Jane's.

If you see yourself in either Jane's or Kisha's story, take heart. Body image and self-esteem are both dynamic processes that can evolve and change throughout your life. A low time in your life doesn't have to last forever. Shedding the self-consciousness and shame of a poor body image can give you the courage to work on other parts of your life such as self-esteem. Remember: It's never too late to start loving your body.

BODY IMAGE AND AGE

Having positive feelings about your body is a definite advantage as you grow older and begin to encounter the unique image problems related to aging. In a society in which the model of feminine beauty is a teenage movie star, older women are in a losing battle. One of the more impossible expectations is that women will remain the same weight throughout life. One Melpomene study asking what weight was "just right" for a 5-foot, 4-inch woman found that 113 was selected for those under 19 and 120-122 for anyone older. This is unrealistic and unhealthy for most older women.

The problem for older women may be a lack of positive depictions of women in their age group. As Martha, a striking, gray-haired woman in our osteoporosis study, remarked, "I have a problem. I don't have any real role models for how I should look or behave." To put yourself in Martha's place, think about the media images that flash before you every day; most are of women under 40. Older women either are invisible or are unbelievably glamorous women such as Elizabeth Taylor, Lena Horne, and Joan Collins. The television show *The Golden Girls,* now in syndication, was one of the few series in which perfect body shape and no wrinkles were not requirements. The show has received excellent ratings which may indicate how eager older women are for positive reflections of themselves.

We don't have much research information that tracks how older women see their bodies. In a current review of all the literature on body image, only six studies included older adults in the sample. Melpomene's studies of older women are among the only sources to which we can turn. These studies indicate that overall, satisfaction with looks increases

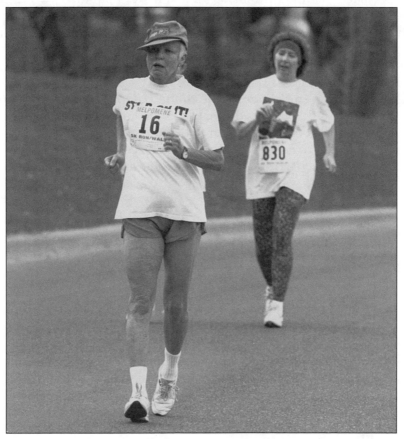

Giving up on the idea that your body is going to stay the same as you grow older probably means that you are not only older, but wiser—and healthier!

with age. In our 1985 membership study, 39 percent of women aged 20-29 believed they looked better than most women, while 87 percent of women over 50 chose that response.

Physical activity seems to boost that positive response even higher. In a follow-up body image questionnaire answered by women in the Melpomene osteoporosis study, 96 percent of the high activity group were generally satisfied with the way they look; this was also true of 76 percent of the medium activity group and 72 percent of the low activity group. Sixty-seven percent of the high activity group were quite satisfied, which was twice as many as the low activity group.

Not only does physical activity favorably influence body image, but it also seems to impact health. Sixty-three percent of the high activity group stated that their health was much better than most, while only 7 percent of the women with a low activity rating chose that response. Ninety-eight percent of the high activity group said they had a feeling of looking strong and healthy, compared with 85 percent of the medium activity group and 57 percent of the low activity group.

In many ways, it is a shame that we don't start feeling better about our bodies at an earlier age. Some of the older women to whom we spoke regretted that they had spent so much time, energy, and money chasing after an idealized version of beauty instead of just celebrating the body they had. As we have seen, our society perpetuates the myth that a woman needs to "improve" herself because she is, presumably, imperfect in some way. Convincing yourself otherwise is a great challenge, but it's worth it.

BECOMING COMFORTABLE WITH THE BODY YOU HAVE

How can you begin to like your body better? The following case studies may give you some ideas for possible changes. Age need not be a barrier.

Gwen began to cross-country ski when she was 63. She had almost abandoned exercise after years of physical activity related both to her job as a part-time physical education instructor and family hiking and biking trips. Subtle changes in both body shape and appetite encouraged her to try something new. "As a kid," she recalled, "I was always active in team sports. It was rare, but I attended a private school where those opportunities were available. I guess I always saw myself as fairly skilled athletically, and it helped me deal with being 5 feet, 11 inches. I also thought that because of my height I would never get fat and out of shape." She laughed. "I have some pictures to show that that wasn't true in my later years. I love skiing," she said, "because it has made me fit again, but most important, it's given me a sense of independence and strength."

Because she had been a fat child, Jenny still thought of herself as fat even when she had become a skinny adult. Competitive running did little to improve her body image. She continued to carefully watch what she ate and rarely consumed more than 1,000 calories per day. After several years of running, her weight stabilized at 105 pounds, low average weight for her 5-foot, 4-inch height. Her efficient body seemed to know when she ate more, and she frequently noted a 3-pound gain after a weekend of heavier eating. Following an injury, Jenny found that her weight began to creep up. Friends convinced her she needed to consume more calories to remain healthy. Jenny now weighs 120 pounds. She still wishes it was easy to eat what she wants to and stay slim, but she has learned to accept her new body shape. When she looks at old pictures she actually thinks she was too thin, but her new perceptions remain vulnerable, and she still needs to be reassured that she really doesn't look fat.

Gwen's and Jenny's stories suggest that change will probably be easier if your body image was positive as a child. It may encourage you to pay attention to your own children's attitudes and perceptions. If you have some concerns about your body image, now might be a good time to try to put these concerns into perspective. Once you have done that, change will be easier.

Check Your Own Perceptions

Think for a moment about the models with whom you usually compare yourself. Is your reference group a fair appraisal of your own fatness and fitness? If you are comparing yourself with television and magazine models, your 17-year-old daughter, or competitive athletes, you are clearly stacking the deck against yourself. Yet, many midlife and older women tell us that they find it hard to accept the weight gain or shift that comes with menopause. Many remember their mothers as soft and slightly overweight. "My mother," says Sarah, "was very happy being seen as 'grandmotherly.' She had a very comfortable lap and a wonderful smile. Even though she might have been overweight on a scale, she remained active and healthy until she died at 87." Sarah wishes that she could feel good about letting her body mellow that way with age. "These days," she says, "a woman is expected to look young and thin until she dies."

Do you have that expectation for yourself and other people? One interesting way to look at body image and decide if you need to work on your own perceptions and goals is to buy a roll of film and take pictures of people of all ages and both sexes. Take your pictures in various public places—a park, a concert, a running race, a baseball game, a shopping center. When you get them developed, look at the expressions on people's faces as well as their external appearance. What kinds of assumptions do you make about these people based on the photos?

Next, look at pictures of yourself; group pictures may be especially useful. Subconsciously, you may have already ranked yourself in size and weight against the rest of your friends and colleagues. Take a good look now at the evidence; are you really fatter than the rest of the group, or is this feeling part of a perception problem? What if you *are* larger than most people? Can you improve your body image without changing your size? Consider concentrating not on a physical comparison but rather on positive individual qualities. In the past 10 years the size acceptance movement has helped many women see that the problem lies in society's judgmental stance on overweight people.

Get Moving

Being or becoming physically active is a great way to improve your body image and boost your confidence in other areas as well. Don't be discouraged if early attempts to play tennis, walk, or bike are not an immediate success. Having a body that "functions" well will definitely increase self-esteem. "Functioning" will, however, have different meanings for different ages, shapes, and abilities. Naturally, the woman who is 60 and has arthritis will not be able to do the same things as the 16-year-old gymnast. The 25-five-year-old athlete who has become quadriplegic as the result of an accident will also have to modify her perspective of what it means to be physically active. Yet, each of us who begins to see what her body can do will find herself more confident in other areas as well.

Keep a Record of Your Progress

If you have problems in some of the areas discussed in this chapter, begin today to change them! Don't say, "I have to watch what I eat," even though it may take years before you don't think that sentence.

Begin to think about things you do well, physically and mentally, and work on those. It may help to make a list of aspects you like about yourself, again both physical and mental qualities, and put it somewhere where you can read it 6 months later. One of the best ways to keep track of your feelings and progress is to start a diary.

Edith had been having problems at work, her relationship with her spouse of 15 years showed signs of strain, and she wasn't sure what was happening. She had read that keeping a journal might be helpful and decided to try to write whenever she was moved to do so. Now, 12 years later, Edith has eight volumes of thoughts and musings. While she is not sure they have ever been responsible for solving major problems, the act of writing things down has often been helpful. About once a year, she takes the time to skim through her journals to see if she can find anything useful or revealing. She is encouraged by the fact that she seems more mellow and is certainly happier with her body (although it's both enlarged and slipped downward!).

For Edith, keeping a personal journal was enough; the act of writing helped her express anger and joy. It helped articulate problems and identify options. Over the years rereading the journal has been both instructive and soothing.

Find People Who Will Nurture You

Samantha, in contrast, doesn't express herself well in writing. She found that talking to her friends was the best way for her to sort through her body and self-image problems. As a runner who was returning to school as a "much older student," she had numerous concerns about fitting in and being successful. One thing that helped her work through these issues was to start a running group with other women who were in the same situation. She noted, "I found that the act of running made me more open in my remarks; as my friendship with that small group of women developed, I was able to discuss things I never would have thought possible."

Seek Professional Help

Some women may wish or need to seek professional advice and help. The following suggestions may help you select the appropriate professional. If possible, find someone who has experience with clients who have body image concerns or problems. It may be worthwhile to talk with one of the clients to gain a better understanding of the professional's perspective and usual methods. Some believe that a change in behaviors leads to a change in attitudes; others prefer to move from attitudes toward changed behaviors; still others, who have a more flexible style, will move in whatever direction works for you.

Once you have identified several nutritionists or psychologists, the next step is to talk with one or two of them on the phone. Look for someone who treats you seriously. Ann Meissner, a psychologist who has been a speaker at numerous Melpomene conferences, suggests that you conduct an interview on the phone, or perhaps in person. This first conversation should do more than answer questions about the process; you should also come away with the feeling that the professional "likes you" and is willing to help you work through your issues. Meissner also says that she seldom recommends that a client see a therapist who is younger. A certain amount of empathy will come from having experienced some things firsthand.

A good professional should be able to help you start accepting your body. If weight loss is part of a sensible program, be sure that you are getting some psychological support as well. Meissner believes that losing weight can markedly change self-concept. In fact, it occasionally comes as a surprise to many people that this change may have negative as well as positive elements.

Remember that the method that the professional prefers may not be a good fit for you. Throughout the process, it will pay for you to evaluate how much progress you feel you are making. If you feel the method is no longer working, perhaps it's time to adjust the approach. Take advantage of the momentum you've already gained to bring you all the way in to home base—safe and feeling good inside your own body.

CELEBRATE THE BODY YOU HAVE

We hope that after reading this chapter, you have some different perceptions about what constitutes a "good" body. Take the quiz on page 33 again. Maybe you would now rank "strong and healthy" above "thin and petite." Maybe you've begun to see your own body more realistically, and begun to appreciate it for its flexibility or muscle tone, rather than haggling over the few extra pounds you've gained this year.

Once you've made friends with your body, you'll need to tend the relationship as natural changes occur. The flat stomach you are proud of in your twenties will soften and grow rounder with age. Your joints may get stiffer, and your running times may get slower. Or, you could become disabled and not be able to run at all anymore. The challenge is to let your standards change along with your body and to congratulate yourself for who you are at that particular moment.

It's a wonderful feeling to be proud of your body. Gaining physical confidence can alter the way you see yourself in the world. For swimmer Diana Nyad, being a physically strong woman makes her feel as if "she owns the earth." At Melpomene, we like to try to imagine what the world would be like if we all ignored the cultural prescriptions for female beauty and began to feel at home in our own bodies. Think of what we could do with all the time and energy we currently spend dieting and "improving" ourselves!

Where to Receive Information About Eating Disorders:

The American Anorexia-Bulimia Association
293 Central Park West #1R
New York, NY 10024
(212) 501-8351

ANAD—National Association of Anorexia Nervosa and
Associated Disorders
P.O. Box 7
Highland Park, IL 60035
(708) 831-3438

ANRED—Anorexia Nervosa and Related Eating Disorders
P.O. Box 5102
Eugene, OR 97405
(503) 344-1144

Center for the Study of Anorexia Nervosa and Bulimia
One West 91st Street
New York, NY 10024
(212) 595-3449

NEDO—National Eating Disorders Organization
6655 South Yale Avenue
Tulsa, OK 74101
(918) 481-4044

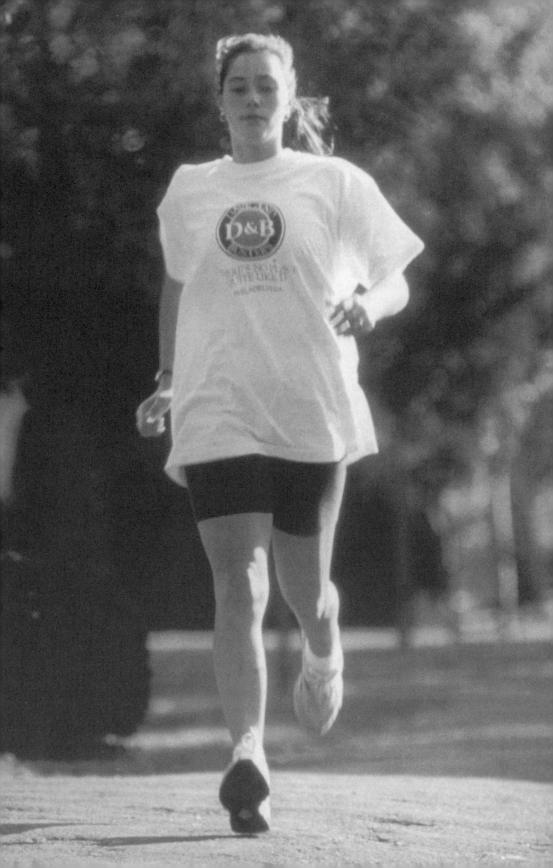

3

How to Get Moving!

With two jobs and two children, Linda feels she lacks the time and energy for regular workouts. Before she had the children, she ran and biked regularly. Now she has let physical activity fall lower on her priority ladder. A friend of Linda's has asked her if she'd be interested in daily early-morning walks of about 2 miles. Linda likes the idea but has never thought of walking as vigorous exercise. Can she really get fit and stay fit if her main physical activity is walking?

While Teri is active sporadically, her greatest obstacle in sticking with a plan seems to be boredom. She takes an occasional aerobics class and became involved in Frisbee golf for about 2 weeks. Teri wants to be in better shape, and she wonders how she can stay committed to a regular routine. She thinks she could stick with a routine if only she enjoyed the activity, so she has been looking for something that is fun and not too demanding, at least at first. What are her best options?

It seems as if the "self-help" book has been with us forever, but actually, the idea of women making their own health and well-being a priority is relatively new. Throughout history, we as women have been expected to take care of everyone else's emotional and physical needs first. The families and communities that we tended assumed that we would always be there, mysteriously able to maintain good health in spite of adverse or stressful conditions. Only rarely did we admit that we were tired or ill. When you consider where we've been, you realize how revolutionary it is for us to suddenly be taking care of ourselves for a change.

For many of us, physical activity has become a major component of this new emphasis on self-care. An unprecedented amount of media attention has hailed exercise as a virtual cure-all for what ails us. And while some of the claims about exercise's beneficial effects are sensationalized, many are indeed true. Even so, some women still don't see physical activity as an answer for them personally.

Because many adult American women were not encouraged to be physically active as children, and have little experience with competition, they are hesitant to try something new. "I'd feel foolish," and "I know I won't be any good," are two of the most frequent responses women make when asked to take tennis lessons or join others for a game of golf. Another central barrier to exercise, identified as the most important by respondents to a Melpomene survey, is a lack of free time. Most women today find that time is precious; making time for yourself is difficult no matter what your age or circumstance.

In Melpomene's experience, most women have a hard time relating to the exercise books that have proliferated along with the fitness boom. They call us to ask, "I know it works for actresses and young, thin, independently wealthy women, but how can physical activity help me feel better? How can I fit it into my already busy schedule? How will I get started? What will keep me motivated?"

BENEFITS OF EXERCISE

For more than a decade Melpomene Institute has been conducting research on its members. In 1990, Melpomene conducted a membership survey of more than 600 women. We asked members to tell us about the best part of regular exercise. Half of the respondents listed physical benefits including more strength, feeling healthier, feeling more fit, sleeping better, weight control, being in shape or condition, and looking good. Mental benefits, including stress reduction, relaxation, time for self, mental and spiritual well-being, better attitude, and improved outlook, were cited as a reason for 40 percent of the respondents.

Some of the aforementioned physical benefits of exercise have been well documented in laboratory tests. The psychological gains are harder to measure, however, and therefore have not been addressed as frequently in research. In our study, women were able to offer direct feedback about the personal growth they had experienced after becoming active. They told us that exercise had changed their lives, personal relationships, and self-esteem. It became apparent that women are exercising not only for a healthier body, but also for the good feelings that go hand in hand with a physically active lifestyle.

Physical Benefits

Most of us know that regular exercise is good for you. But did you know that some of the benefits of a regular physical activity program include lowering your risk of having a heart attack, strengthening your bones, and decreasing your risk for diabetes?

Exercise decreases your risk of heart disease by strengthening your heart. Physical activity can also lower your risk of heart disease by increasing HDL, the good kind of cholesterol that actually hunts for harmful cholesterol in the body, taking it to the liver where it is burned up. Regular exercise can increase your aerobic capacity, which is the amount of oxygen your lungs can breathe in and utilize. Physical

The Best Part of Regular Exercise

The best part of regular exercise according to more than 600 respondents of the 1990 Melpomene membership study:

Physical benefits	49.9%
Mental benefits	39.6%
It generally feels good	37.5%
Positive self-image	17.4%
Feels good afterwards	8.8%
Enjoyment, fun	4.6%
Training, maintaining fitness	3.7%
Being outdoors, environment	3.3%

activity can also lower your risk of having high blood pressure, diabetes, and breast cancer. Weight-bearing exercise has also been shown to increase bone mass and actually retard or reverse the normal loss of bone mineral content. Likewise, exercise has been instrumental for many people in weight control.

Improved Self-Esteem

Improved self-image and confidence have been frequently mentioned as benefits of physical activity throughout Melpomene's research. The confidence that comes from being able to engage in a sport successfully is a huge boost to self-esteem. The definition of success varies. For some women, it means swimming for 10 minutes nonstop, and for others, it means running a marathon.

Women also told us that they were proud to be participating or competing in a sport that society had at one time considered inappropriate for women. Like most of us, they had been programmed to believe that there were certain physical activities that they shouldn't or couldn't do because of their gender. Women who defy these damaging stereotypes tend to gain confidence and a better self-image. Active women tell us:

"I feel better about myself—my overall appearance. I have more confidence in myself, more self-assurance, and a better body image. I have something to talk about—myself."

"I have a better self-image, self-esteem. It's easier to love others when you love yourself."

"My improved self-image has improved my family relationships."

"I feel better about my body. I am more outgoing and confident; I take more risks."

A Stress Reliever

With the lack of time to exercise being cited as a major obstacle for women, it would seem that trying to fit a workout into a packed schedule would further complicate an already stressful lifestyle. However, this is not the case. In the 1990 study of Melpomene members, women reported that physical activity was beneficial in relieving stress. Many stated that exercise was the best means they had found for relieving the day's stress and tensions. After working out, women described an after-exercise "glow"—the feeling of more energy and well-being. Some said that the way they felt afterwards was their main reason for exercising.

"I'm more relaxed."

"The best part of regular exercise is the feeling of exhilaration and well-being; always feeling energetic."

"Being in shape gives a feeling of well-being and confidence to take on challenges in all parts of life. Certainly I handle stress better."

"Exercise is very important to me as a means of stress management."

We all live with stress in varying degrees and forms throughout our lives. Our bodies are designed to live with a certain amount of stress as part of basic survival. Hundreds of years ago, it was the stress response that allowed humans to run for the hills when a saber-toothed tiger stalked them. Today's demands are different, but the body still tries to protect itself, exhibiting behaviors that can take the form of shivering with the cold, to intense anger and fear.

Although a lifestyle with minimal stress sounds ideal, it would be very dull. Stress has some very positive aspects, among them:

- *Challenge.* We all need a certain amount of challenge in our lives, whether in the form of giving a speech, swimming in a timed event, or receiving a hard-earned promotion. It is the challenges we encounter that keep us stimulated.
- *Change.* Although change can be a very strong stressor, it enables us to grow. With every challenge or change, we become stronger individuals, more able to cope.
- *Variety.* A variety of life situations and challenges is essential to living to your full potential. Without variety, again, our lives become dull and boring.

When a person experiences stress, the nervous and endocrine systems are activated, producing the "fight or flight," or alarm, response. These responses are meant to deal with short-term situations (such as getting away from the saber-tooth). Over the long term, the body's physiology becomes altered by these continually overstimulated and overactivated organs, causing the organs to wear down or become diseased. Stress can also interfere with the normal functioning of the immune system. It is believed that lowered immunity from stress is a major cause of colds, infection, and even cancer. Thus, it is ironic that the same responses that were intended to facilitate our survival can make us ill if we continually experience them over a long period of time.

A healthy, well-conditioned body is at the foundation of all stress-coping strategies. For this reason, many people use exercise as their primary source of stress reduction. There are several reasons why exercise works so well. First, vigorous physical activity is a natural outlet for your body when it is in the "fight or flight" stage of arousal. Exercise allows you to work off that adrenaline rush, and afterwards, it allows your body to return to its pre-stress state of equilibrium.

Exercise also allows for periods of relaxed concentration, similar to meditation. This transcendent experience has been called a "runner's high," but can occur in any form of physical activity. Endorphins, painkilling chemicals released in the brain, are partly responsible for the runner's high. Endorphins have also been associated with increased pain tolerance, reduced anxiety, and improved appetite control. Another benefit of physical activity is the recreation factor, or simply taking the time out from a busy day to enjoy a pleasurable activity.

Nutrition and Stress

Even though most of us don't think of proper nutrition as a stress-reduction technique, there are ways that we compound our stress through poor nutrition. An obvious example of this is high caffeine intake. Caffeine, a stimulant found in coffee, black tea, colas, and chocolate, chemically induces a "fight or flight" response in your body. Therefore, if you are feeling stressed during the day, caffeine will only make matters worse.

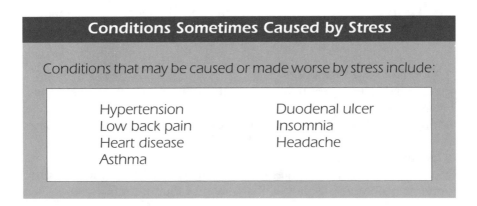

Conditions Sometimes Caused by Stress

Conditions that may be caused or made worse by stress include:

Hypertension	Duodenal ulcer
Low back pain	Insomnia
Heart disease	Headache
Asthma	

Lower Your Stress Through Nutrition

- Eat a good breakfast. A sugary pastry and a cup of coffee do not meet your body's needs for a good breakfast.
- Eat foods high in B vitamins and calcium. If you are under a lot of stress, these nutrients will be even more important.
- Eat a wide variety of foods to ensure that you are getting enough nutrients.
- Eat four or five small meals a day. Frequent eating avoids stress associated with hunger, and keeps blood sugar even.
- Take the time to eat. Eat slowly, and enjoy the relaxation that comes from eating good food in unhurried surroundings.

Sugar can also affect how you feel. When you eat foods high in sugar, your blood sugar level shoots up, giving you a boost of energy for a short period of time. However, your pancreas produces insulin to counter the sugar in your blood, depressing your blood sugar level to a point lower than before. This low blood sugar can cause dizziness, irritability, depression, shaking, nausea, and hunger pangs that may prompt you to have another sweet snack.

Some people drink alcohol as a form of stress reduction. However, alcohol is a depressant, which slows certain functions in some parts of the brain. Alcohol can also irritate the gastrointestinal tract, cause a hangover, and inhibit sleep. Overall, this does not seem to be a healthy or practical way to reduce stress.

Social Benefits

"It definitely has increased my social sphere and number of friends."

"I've met lots of good friends through the sport of orienteering."

"Physical activity has allowed me a vent for frustration and allowed me fellowship and being part of a group."

Social interaction associated with exercise has been a key psychological benefit for many of the Melpomene members who we have studied. They state that sport gave them a chance to meet new people, as well as a way to share a common activity with old friends. An interesting pattern emerged in women's comments about the effects of exercise on their relationships. Many women noted that they had developed more tolerance and understanding toward others as a result of feeling better about themselves. Many relationships had improved or been sparked as a result of their new lifestyle. A surprising number had met their spouse or partner through a shared sport.

At the same time, some active women noticed that they no longer had as much time for sedentary friends. This may be because their new exercise programs were keeping them busy, or simply because they now had less in common with friends who had different lifestyle priorities.

"A shared activity with my spouse makes it more enjoyable; makes sure we both get our exercise each day."

"My husband, mother, and friends are very proud of my success in weight loss and physical abilities. I have more energy when I keep my weight down and get some regular activity."

"Since I feel better about myself, I deal with people and situations better. I have a firmer base."

Challenging Yourself

Finally, some women in our studies said that they valued physical activity because it offered them the chance to challenge themselves in the physical arena. Through sport, they could set goals for themselves and experience the sense of accomplishment that is so often lacking in our normal work and home lives. Regardless of your age or ability, the chance to watch yourself improve—to break your own records—can positively affect your life.

If you have basically been sedentary, the first challenge is to decide that physical activity and the lifestyle changes that usually accompany it are worth the effort. Deciding to start and sticking with it may be two different things, however. In short-term exercise programs, the dropout rate is as high as 40 percent. In longer-term commitments (8 weeks or more), that figure jumps to 75 percent.

CHOOSING AN EXERCISE PROGRAM

If you are not currently active, or wish to explore ways to increase or diversify your level of physical activity, try filling out the personal profile below. Rereading it will give you some insights into your knowledge of and attitudes toward exercise.

A Personal Profile

1. How many hours per day do you work? (time that you do not consider leisure)
2. How many hours per day are you basically sitting at work?
3. How many flights of stairs do you climb in an average week?
4. How many blocks do you walk in an average week?
5. How many hours per day do you spend doing house-keeping chores such as cooking and cleaning?
6. How many hours (or minutes) per day do you have that are "yours"?
   What do you do during this time? (read, watch TV, knit, exercise)
7. How interesting is physical activity to you? (Be honest!)
8. What would be your main aims in beginning a physical activity program?
9. Think about your current schedule: What options do you have to fit in one-half hour or one hour per day of exercise?
10. What is your energy level at this time of day?
11. Are you more likely to exercise alone, with a friend, or in a class situation?
12. What are some realistic goals regarding physical activity for the next three weeks?
13. Try to list some goals for the next three months.

Finding Time

Defining the number of hours you work is sometimes quite enlightening. We've used this questionnaire in many of our seminars, and invariably, women have been astounded by their own answers. "Well," sighed one, "no wonder I have such trouble finding time to exercise. I'm actually working a 15-hour day!" This women is a public health administrator who works 8 hours a day at the office and frequently brings home a briefcase of work that she tackles for 2 hours in the evening. In addition she is the mother of three young children who finds that the hours from 6 p.m. until they are in bed are filled with household responsibilities. On the other hand, one woman who has recently returned to school to complete a graduate degree found that for the first time she can actually attend classes and complete her studying in 8 hours. "Until I filled out the profile, however," she remarked, "I was still living as I did when I worked full-time and went to school. I realized I needed to figure out where the rest of my time was going."

More and more of us spend the better part of our days in work that is sedentary. Many of us have desk jobs that require little physical energy or effort. Most likely, we work in an environment where it is easier to take the elevator than use the stairs. Often, employees in these buildings would be hard pressed to say where the stairway is located. Think of how inactive we've become in contrast to our ancestors who lived when farm, factory, and housework all required standing, lifting, and moving.

Because we are rarely forced to incorporate physical activity into our daily patterns, finding time to do so on a structured basis is often difficult.

> "I need to relax when I get home; going for a run would be ridiculous."

> "What do you mean, take a break before dinner? If I did that, no one would eat until 7, and that just wouldn't work."

To the people making these statements, the obstacles they list are real and seemingly insurmountable. If your answer to question 6 (How many hours per day do you have that are "yours"?) is low, and you really treasure this time to read or watch TV, then it may be very hard to psychologically make the decision to begin exercising. Yet, there is good evidence that if you can convince yourself that physical activity is important, you may indeed find a way to eliminate the obstacles. People who are not yet in the habit of exercising need a lot of evidence before they will believe that taking a brief, brisk walk or a leisurely jog will leave them more relaxed than sitting down with a drink or the evening paper. But scientific and practical observation proves this is true. Ask any elementary school teacher who faces a classroom of kids in the afternoon: Students are always more alert and easier to teach after an active recess. After a lunch with no recess, the same students are more likely to feel like napping.

Choosing the Right Activity

Carving out a time for exercise in an already busy day is a real problem for most of us. That's why your answer to question 7 (How interesting is physical activity to you?) is so important. Many of us can think of physical activities that are not interesting to us at all. To some people, aerobic dance is ridiculous, while others think running looks like a modern-day form of torture. Naturally, choosing those activities would be self-defeating for these people; they'd have little incentive to overcome the inertia of their daily routine. One key to choosing a physical activity or exercise program is to list four or five activities that sound like fun and then find a sport that combines the best of these. Think of an activity that gave you pleasure when you were young, or that has intrigued you as an adult. "I'd really like to try racquetball," said one woman, "because it looks like fun."

Next, you might want to consider your answer to the eighth question (What would be your main aims in starting an exercise program?). If

What Do You Like to Do?

List physical activities that interest you.

1.

2.

3.

4.

5.

6.

your main aim is cardiovascular fitness, you should consider walking, running, vigorous biking, or swimming. Other programs will also qualify if you do them at least three times a week for a duration of 30 minutes at 80 percent of your heart rate.

If, however, your main aim is to look and feel better, you may be able to start at a lower level with sports that can be less demanding. Playing doubles tennis twice a week with other beginners may not improve your fitness level at first, but in time, as you become a better player, you may want to play more often or play a more vigorous game. (On the other hand, you might thoroughly enjoy your relaxed, nonstressful games and never make any great changes in intensity. That's completely up to you.)

You may not be able to identify one physical activity that you have been eager to try, or you may not feel that you have time to even think about a new activity. In that case just adding physical activity to your daily routine might be the answer for you. Some women have found that regularly parking an extra half-mile from work and walking to and from the office can make a difference in the entire day. Others find that making an effort to use the stairs, as opposed to taking the elevator, keeps them more alert and helps keep them going. There may be other ways you can think of for incorporating physical activity into your daily routine. Be creative and have fun.

Perhaps you want some variety and excitement in your exercise program. If you have primarily been a runner or a softball player for most of your life, this may be the time to look at diversifying your activities. You may want to consider something entirely new such as horseback riding, cross-country skiing, or golf.

Your choice of activity will also depend on your schedule and your need to be alone or with people.

Lisa works with people all day. She frequently chairs meetings in the morning and spends all afternoon with clients. Her friend Chris urged her to join the local fitness club so that they could exercise together at the end of the day. Since Lisa was having trouble motivating herself to exercise, she decided to give it a try. The courts and track were well maintained, and the club was convenient, yet within 2 weeks Lisa was ready to quit. What she hadn't realized was that the crowds that used the facility at the same time she did would put her on edge, especially after a full day of people contact. Instead, Lisa decided to tune up her old bike and strike out on her own.

Scheduling

Scheduling is particularly crucial where jobs and young children are involved. In a Melpomene Institute study of women who ran or swam during their pregnancies, a large number said that they exercised less and less after their child was born. One of the major reasons was not being able to find anyone to baby-sit. It's also hard for many women who work outside the home to justify leaving a child in day care for an extra hour or so at the end of a day. For that reason many chose to exercise before others were awake. Jane frequently is at the YWCA pool by 6 a.m. "It's my only choice," she says, "and while I almost resented it at first, I've discovered it's a great way to start the day." It's not as easy to find a partner for tennis at that hour, but groups of walkers and bikers are also known to meet, exercise, shower, and be at work by 8 a.m. Scheduling may pose more problems if you decide to set a time-consuming goal such as running a marathon or riding a century (a 100-mile bike ride).

What happens if your body is not ready to exercise at the hour that's most convenient for you? If you're like Mary, you wake up feeling as if you are 59 instead of 36. Mary has some mild arthritis which bothers her only early in the morning. She finds that lunchtime or after work, though they may not be as convenient, are better times for her to exercise.

It is clear from these brief examples that choosing an exercise program can be more complex than promoters would have us believe. The ads look great: young, attractive, thin people swimming and hitting tennis balls as if there are no hassles involved. While most people who are serious about physical exercise know that it's not always convenient or easy, they are also the first to try to convince you to give it a try.

HOW TO START

For many women, just deciding to become physically active can be the biggest hurdle to overcome. Some women are able to begin by just walking out the front door to a regular walking or running program. If you are like most women, however, there are many practical considerations to make before starting. Remember, though, that your situation is unique—and only you can determine what will work given your lifestyle, time constraints, and level of commitment. We offer the following suggestions and encouragement to anyone trying to become more active.

Consider Your Health

Each woman needs to take stock of her health and medical history before entering an exercise program of any kind. Some general guidelines established by the American College of Sports Medicine (ACSM) suggest that if you are a man under age 40 or a woman under age 50 with no signs, symptoms, or history of cardiovascular problems or other risk factors, such as diabetes or hypertension, you need not get a medical checkup. Currently the ACSM is moving toward the use of a seven-point questionnaire to help adults assess their own readiness for increased physical activity.

You may, however, choose to check with your health-care provider if you have concerns about your health or the exercise program you are about to undertake. We encourage you to make an appointment if you have an underlying medical condition such as cardiovascular disease, hypertension, or diabetes, or if you have a family history of any of these conditions.

Other health factors that you will want to take into consideration before starting to exercise include any chronic conditions or illnesses, disabilities, or previous injuries. These shouldn't stop you from being physically active, but you should consider them when choosing your sport or the kind of equipment you will use.

Choose the Right Physical Activity for You

There are many factors to consider when you choose an activity. The most important is that it should be fun. If you are not enjoying your exercise program or the sport you choose, you will not continue to do it. Ideally, you will be able to find a few activities that you enjoy well enough to keep you active throughout your lifetime.

Your age might be a factor in the activity you choose. Our 1990 membership survey of more than 600 women showed us that favored activities do seem to change with age. Running, for example, was extremely popular with women in their fifties and younger, but lost its allure for women in their sixties and above. In our 1984-85 survey, golf became more popular as women's age increased. In 1990, however, responses showed that golf has increased in popularity for younger women as well. The percentages of women golfers were about even for women in their thirties through their eighties. While some women continued working out with weights into their fifties and sixties, their numbers generally dropped with age. Aerobics or calisthenics, however, remained popular for women in their fifties, sixties, and seventies. Racquet sports, team sports, and skating dropped to almost zero for women past the age of 50.

While age is not necessarily a barrier to any activity, it seems that as the women in our study grew older, they gravitated toward different sports that fit their changing needs. This change in choice of activity with age reminds us once again that sport is a treat for the self, and should be a source of enjoyment or relaxation.

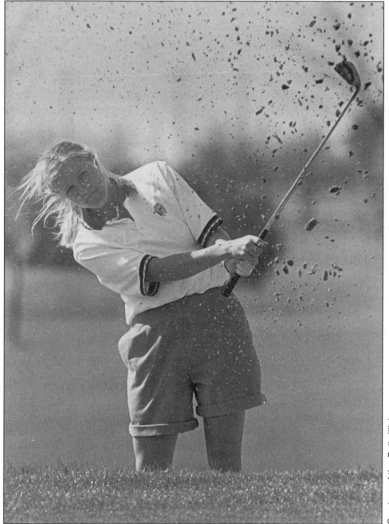

Courtesy of the *Daily Illini*

Unlike most other sports, golf is equally popular among women of all ages.

The time you have for physical activity may also influence your choice of activity. If your time is limited, as is the case for many of us, you may choose a daily activity that can be done in a fairly short amount of time, and save more time-consuming activities for the weekends. For example, you may take a walk each day during the week and plan to canoe for several hours on the weekend.

A full calendar of responsibilities with family or friends and/or work may force you to come up with creative ways to squeeze in workouts during the week. This may mean a tennis game during lunch hour or trading child care with another physically active friend. If you have younger children, look for a health club that offers child care. Once they get older, your kids may enjoy a swim or dribbling the basketball at the Y while you attend exercise class.

Your environment, including climate, community, and available facilities, can also affect your choice of physical activity. A northern climate may not seem like an obvious deterrent to your biking program in May, but just wait until December and January roll around. You may be forced to switch to another sport for the winter, or may decide to find a facility where you can exercise indoors during the coldest days.

The community in which you live may also shape the activity you choose. If you live in a large city, it may take longer to get to safe, wide-open roads than it would if you lived in a rural setting. Some rural settings, however, may not offer the kind of equipment or facilities you need for your chosen sport. Considerations such as these can be especially crucial if you travel a lot. Finding an alternate activity that you can "take with you" might be to your advantage.

For almost any activity that needs an actual facility such as a pool, court, or weight room, you will need to spend some time shopping for a site that will suit your needs. Some things you'll want to consider before joining are the initiation and monthly fees, the financial stability of the club, the number of members, the equipment available for your activity, locker and shower facilities, the instructors' qualifications, the hours, and the location. If the club is far from your home, try to imagine yourself getting home from work and then getting back in the car or onto public transportation to commute to your club. Would it be a deterrent?

Many physical activities don't require the use of a facility, but almost all require some special equipment or clothing. This expense, be it large or small, may influence your decision to get involved in an activity. For example, if you were to choose a walking program, you'd need only a good pair of shoes. If you want to start cycling, on the other hand, the start-up costs would certainly be higher. We recommend that you list the clothing, equipment, and facility costs associated with your sport before deciding to make a firm commitment. Also, consider borrowing or renting equipment instead of buying until you are sure you like the activity. Once you've tried it out, you'll also have a better idea of what style of equipment suits you best. One word of caution: Equipment that doesn't fit can unnecessarily discourage you and even cause injury.

Finally, before you undertake a new exercise program, do some soul searching to find out what kind of a participant you'll be. Are you likely to continue a program without group support, or will you need the camaraderie of an organized class? Will you participate on the hottest or coldest days of the year, or do you need an indoor alternative? Are you bored easily? Do you need several different activities to keep you involved? Knowing what motivates and excites you will be important a few months down the road, when the novelty of the sport has worn off, and you might be tempted to stop exercising.

Have a Plan

Writing down what you need before you go to the grocery store always seems to speed the trip and keeps you from buying items you don't need. In the same way, an exercise plan is a good idea when you are beginning to be physically active. A plan might be to walk around the block every day for a week, with a goal of being able to finish the walk without feeling tired. Whatever your ambitions are, a plan will provide you with a sensible program and will help you stay committed to that program.

There are several ways to go about finding the right plan for yourself in the activity you choose. Health clubs or the local YWCA offer classes in many activities from aerobics to swimming to weight lifting. There are also many clubs formed by people who like to get together to share their sport. The best place to find out about these clubs is at a local store that sells sports equipment. For example, if you are trying to hook up with a women's cycling group, you might try asking at a bike store. Also, many newspapers carry a column in their Sunday sports section listing club information and activities. Members of these clubs can give you tips as well as encouragement as you become accustomed to exercise.

Books can also be a valuable source of information when you're setting up a plan. There are two types of books that offer advice on exercise plans. One kind offers a very specific, day-by-day plan that you can follow easily. The other is more general, offering enough information for you to make your own program. Remember, however, that you will not get feedback from a book if you have specific questions or problems once you begin.

You may not need or want any outside direction. Your goal—to walk three days a week, or to take tennis lessons—may be something you can do quite independently. Sometimes, however, having a friend know about, or share, that goal can be very helpful. Ellen and Frances insist they would not have succeeded in their goal of becoming more physically active without each other. Ellen asked Frances one day if she would be interested in walking a mile or so several days a week. Frances agreed and remarked that she had been thinking about getting more exercise ever since she retired. The critical decision, although they didn't realize it at the time, was to meet on a street corner midway between their homes. "The first day, it rained," remembers Frances. "I sat by my phone waiting for Ellen to call to say she wanted to cancel." Ellen of course was waiting for Frances to be the first to call. Since neither of them wanted to be the first to break the plan, each went out in the mild rain. "The secret," says Ellen, "was the corner. It meant that we were serious about walking. If we had met at one of our homes, I'm sure there would have been days when we would have stayed in and had a cup of coffee instead."

Go Slowly

Once you have convinced yourself that you will be physically active, you are probably eager to get started. Hold onto that enthusiasm; you may need it in a few months when time pressures tempt you to quit. Right now, however, our advice is to go slowly. Overdoing physical activity in the early stages of a program is an invitation to burnout and injury. There will be many opportunities to push yourself, but right now, taking it easy will help you to stay fresh and committed to your new activity.

Stick With It!

Promise yourself a minimum amount of time to try your new program. Eight weeks is a good length to give you an idea of whether this is the right plan or activity for you. Less than five or six weeks is not enough time to make a fair judgment. Also, the longer you keep with a plan, the more the activity becomes a habit and a regular part of your life.

There will be days when you don't feel like working out. That's OK; we all have those days. Remember, you are making a major change in your life, and it may not be easy. Some small rewards might help you

Tips for Beginning Exercisers

Martha Stoll Albertson, an exercise physiologist at The Marsh, A Center for Health and Balance, in Minnetonka, Minnesota, offers some tips to help you get the most from an exercise class:

- Wear blinders into your class. Concentrate on what is safe and healthy for you. Don't compete with others; every individual has her own fitness abilities, and trying to live up to others may be harmful to yourself.
- The old adage "no pain, no gain" can be a dangerous one. Your exercise class should not leave you in pain.
- Start your exercise program gradually. It pays to take beginning classes at first so you can get the hang of the routines; not being able to keep up with the class because you're not familiar with the basic moves is frustrating.
- Establish goals, don't make any excuses, exercise with a friend, create a purpose for your exercise, and above all make it fun! The end product should be a stronger, healthier, more flexible and vital you.

stick to your plan on those days when exercise is particularly tough. (You'll find more on staying motivated in the next section.)

Have Fun!

Again, it's important that you are having fun in your exercise program. There are many tricks to keep yourself motivated, but if the activity is not initially fun for you to do, you will not stick with it. You may have to try a few different sports until you find one or two that you really enjoy. Don't give up—physical activity is fun!

STAYING MOTIVATED

Perhaps one of the hardest parts of regular physical activity is staying motivated so that you exercise regularly. Often boredom or increased time constraints are enough of a roadblock to make you stop exercising altogether.

As part of our 1990 membership survey, we asked respondents: "What do you consider the worst part of regular physical activity?" Their replies were diverse, but the overall theme was the same: The biggest challenge is to stay motivated enough to do physical activity regularly.

"It's difficult trying to find time for exercise—trying to prioritize and figuring out what to leave out."

"Finding the mental discipline is the hardest part."

"Getting my bones out of bed and out the door is the worst part."

"The toughest thing is deciding to do it each day."

". . . boredom . . ."

". . . bad weather . . ."

We also asked respondents in the membership survey to rank which obstacles were most likely to keep them from exercising. Specifically we asked, *In the past five years, what obstacles have you experienced to being physically active?* As you can see by the chart on the next page, time is the largest barrier for many women trying to maintain an active lifestyle.

With all these barriers to regular physical activity, you might wonder how so many women manage to overcome the obstacles and remain motivated. Deep-down faith in the results helps, but that's not always enough to rouse us from our recliners. Following are some tactics and ideas you might try if you are finding yourself with more than your share of excuses about why you shouldn't get out there and do your activity.

Do It With Someone Else

Many of the women in our survey said that one of the best parts of physical activity is the chance to exercise with friends or family members, as well as the chance to meet new friends. There are several ways to find people who share your interests. Talk about your sport at work, at church, or wherever you find yourself; eventually you are bound to bump into someone who shares your enthusiasm and has been looking for a partner. If you're interested in taking up a new activity, you could create a built-in partner by asking a friend to take lessons with you.

Our Reasons for Not Being Active

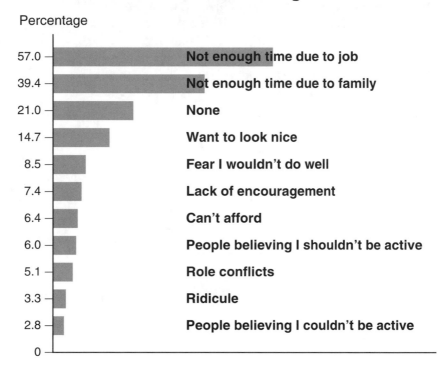

Percentage

57.0	Not enough time due to job
39.4	Not enough time due to family
21.0	None
14.7	Want to look nice
8.5	Fear I wouldn't do well
7.4	Lack of encouragement
6.4	Can't afford
6.0	People believing I shouldn't be active
5.1	Role conflicts
3.3	Ridicule
2.8	People believing I couldn't be active
0	

Make a Contract With Yourself

Some women find that putting a plan down on paper makes it more concrete. You may wish to write a simple contract (like the one shown on page 110) stating how you plan to incorporate physical activity into your life and post it somewhere where you'll see it every day—on a bathroom mirror or refrigerator, for example. The contract is really a commitment you are making to yourself to become physically active.

Try a Change

If you find yourself bored with your workout, try a change. It doesn't have to be big; you can alter your route, work out at a different time, or, if you live in the north country, do your sport indoors in the winter. For some women, changing the structure of their workout can add freshness. For example, if you are swimming a mile in the pool every other day, throwing in some sets of fast laps, arms only, or kicking only, may make your mile feel like a new workout.

Fitness Contract

I promise to incorporate _____ hours of physical activity into my week because: (list as many reasons as you want)

I promise to do this by:

_____
Sign your contract here

Perhaps you need to switch or add a new sport to your physical activity program. A day or two a week on your bike or in the pool can perk up a stale running schedule. Also, seasonal changes offer many opportunities for change in your program. Winter sports such as cross-county skiing or snowshoeing can give you ample exercise while enhancing your overall conditioning. Swimming, aerobics, or walking around a track can also be substituted when it is too hot to run or play tennis outdoors. By treating yourself to something new, you get to try other sports or different variations of your own sport to see what works, what you like, and what you may want to add to your regular program in the future.

Give Yourself a Reward

When you are feeling sluggish, offer yourself a treat for completing your workout. You might promise yourself a long, hot bath; a massage; a new piece of sports clothing; or whatever else really pleases you. This is your way of patting yourself on the back. Not only will you feel proud of yourself for having completed your workout, but you'll have a reward to look forward to as well. Some people have found that keeping a chart and rewarding your progress with gold stars, just like the ones you got in kindergarten, is a great way to reward yourself and keep track of just how far you've progressed.

Set Goals

Goals can be wonderful incentives to continue with an exercise program. Your goal can be keeping with it for a set number of months, obtaining a certain level of endurance or skill, or even a future competition in

Creative Goals

Be creative when setting exercise goals. You might do one or more of the following:

- Give yourself a reward for sticking with your program for a month (or whatever time span is realistic for you). A reward should be something you like but might not ordinarily do for yourself—such as getting a massage, obtaining tickets to an upcoming concert, or buying a new piece of clothing.
- Choose an event to work toward. This could be an upcoming hiking trip that keeps you on your walking plan, a bike tour next summer, or an upcoming race or event in your sport.
- Pay yourself. Put a dollar in a jar for each day you stick with your plan. After you have $50 in the jar (or whatever amount you specify) take the money out and spend it on (or save it toward) something you really want—for example, a new bike, workout outfit, or night out.
- Figure out the mileage to another city in your state (or another state) that you would like to visit. Each day that you run, bike, walk, or swim, add up your mileage until you have imaginarily reached that city.
- Make a deal with yourself. You don't have to do your complete workout—but you do have to start it. Once you get started you'll usually end up doing the whole workout.
- If you are starting out in a new sport, make your goal to get better at it—improve your bicycling skills, work toward a more challenging aerobics class, or learn a new cross-country skiing technique.

your activity. A word of caution here: Be realistic with your goals. The goals you set should be obtainable for you, yet feel like an achievement. You don't want to set marks so high that you will never be able to obtain them; this sets you up for failure and works against your efforts to stay motivated.

Get Into or Out of Competition

If you are competitive in your sport, give yourself a break and do your sport just for fun. Without the pressure of upcoming competitions, you'll be able to recapture the sense of fun that first attracted you to the activity. On the other hand, if you have never competed in your sport, you may want to set your sights on an upcoming event or competition. If you are not feeling competitive, there are often events held in various activities that are noncompetitive gatherings. Organized bike rides, fun runs, and exhibitions in various sports fit this category. An upcoming event in your sport may give you a tangible reason for keeping up with your physical activity program.

Try Something Completely New

Have you always wanted to snowshoe? Do you wonder what canoeing is like? Have you been itching to try a mountain bike? Now is the time to give these and other interesting activities a try. These days, you can rent almost any piece of sporting equipment imaginable. You may want to get a friend or a group of friends to try a new activity with you. You have nothing to lose and everything to gain—you may end up with a new favorite pastime!

Set Up a Home Fitness Center

A home fitness center does not have to be a weight room and exercise studio. It can be as simple as an aerobics tape and a good mat or a stationary exercise bike. The convenience of a home fitness center might be your first choice for fitting exercise into a busy day. Perhaps for you, home equipment can be a backup for those rainy days or the days when you don't have the time to get out of the house. A 10-second commute to your basement will leave you plenty of time to work out, even when you have less than an hour to exercise. Your home equipment might also be an alternative to your regular routine, just for the sake of variety!

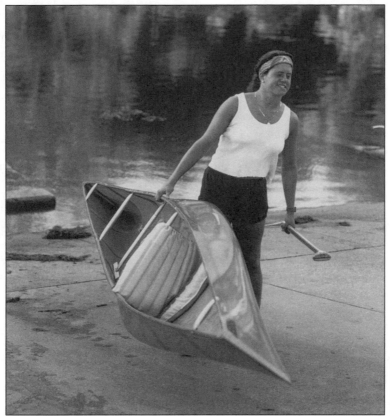

Looking for an activity to love? Something to get you moving? Why not try something new?

© David R. Barnes

Avoid Becoming Obsessive About Exercise

For many women, exercise can bring on feelings of compulsion, with subsequent guilt if they skip a day or want to stop for a while. Some of the women in the Melpomene Institute membership survey mentioned this obsession with exercise as a negative part of being active.

"It can become so important that it begins to assume too much priority."

"The worst part of exercise is the pressure to do it regularly and the disappointment on the days when I just can't discipline myself to do it."

"Exercise can be obsessively burdensome at times."

"Having guilt feelings if you miss a day is a negative."

"I tend to become so obsessed that I risk injury from over-doing it."

Experts in the area of sports psychology debate the issue of whether physical activity is an addiction and, if so, whether it is a positive or a negative addiction. Certainly, we all may have days when we push ourselves out the door to exercise, or feel disappointed in ourselves for having missed a workout. If exercise begins to bring about strong obsessive feelings, however, it may be time to take a break or switch physical activities.

Review Your Progress

Keep an informal journal or jot notes on a calendar so that you can look back at what you were doing 6 months ago, or even when you first started to exercise. Your progress will surprise you and give you a reason to pat yourself on the back. Also, when you see how far you've come, it will be tougher to quit your program from lack of motivation. Your progress and milestones, however large or small, are cause to celebrate!

Build Fitness Into Other Areas of Your Life

If you find yourself without the time or motivation to do your regular workout, look for creative ways to turn your everyday activities into pulse-quickening exercise. For example, leave your car in the drive-way and ride your bike or walk to the store. Turn walking the dog into an aerobic event. If you are homebound with children, build some activity around exercise, such as a soccer game or a walk in the park. Some household chores can give you the benefits of aerobic exercise without taking the time to change into sweats or drive to the gym; possibilities include vigorous spring cleaning, shoveling snow, gardening, and doing yard work.

Take Some Time Off

Sluggishness and a lack of desire to exercise can be signs that you are doing more than you should, either mentally or physically. Your body may be telling you to take a break, or at least to back off for a while.

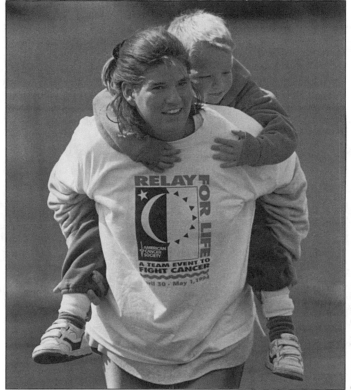

Courtesy of the *Daily Illini*

There are hundreds of ways to make exercise fun—sometimes for more than one of you!

When it's time to start exercising again, your body will also let you know. You will find yourself missing your exercise and wanting to move. Taking a break can bring a sense of novelty and enthusiasm back to your workouts.

AVOIDING INJURY

Becoming injured is a very real concern for many physically active women. Throughout Melpomene research, active women and girls have said that injuries and aches and pains were one of the worst parts of regular exercise.

"I'm injury prone these days—my knee isn't healing."

"The worst part of exercise is having to lay off because of injuries."

"One year ago I sustained tibia stress fractures. I am still recovering from this injury and have to take it easy."

"I have sore legs from concrete and pavement."

Some injuries, especially those from overuse, can be avoided with common sense. Although we all overdo it at some time or other, it is important to take care of our most important piece of equipment—our bodies!

Here are some guidelines Melpomene offers to help women avoid injury:

1. Warm up before you exercise. Warm up by walking around the block, taking a slow run, doing some jumping jacks, anything—just get your blood flowing. Then, before you start really moving your body, take time to stretch. Stretching loosens the muscles you are about to use and increases your range of motion. Inflexible, "cold" muscles are more prone to injury from pulls and strains. Stretching should be a permanent part of your program, not just a quick fix if you think you are becoming injured.

2. Start your physical activity slowly. By starting slowly, you are allowing your body to warm up, your muscles to loosen, and your heart rate and breathing to gradually accelerate.

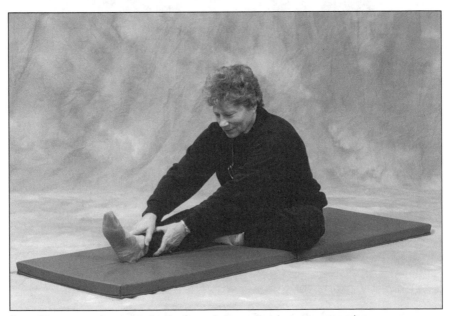

Stretch your major muscles before doing any vigorous exercise.

3. Slow down and cool off after exercise. Walking or doing some light stretching is a good way to end your activity. Cooling down allows your heart rate and breathing to return to normal (pre-exercise) levels. Also, stretching after your workout will help you to avoid muscle soreness.

4. Drink plenty of water! This might seem obvious on hot, humid summer days, but it is important to remember all year long. Before you begin your physical activity, make sure that you are completely hydrated. After you complete exercising, drink at least one glass of water, whether or not you feel thirsty. If you are exercising in hot weather, drinking large amounts of liquids is the best way to help your body cool itself. If you fail to drink enough during extended exercise in hot weather, you can become dehydrated, causing heat stroke or heat exhaustion. Some danger signals are:

- Light-headedness
- Dizziness
- Clamminess
- Lack of perspiration
- Shivering
- Feeling cold

If you or someone you are with should experience any of these symptoms in hot weather, get to a shady or cool spot immediately, and seek medical help. Overheating can be life threatening!

Experts disagree as to what is the best liquid for athletes to drink. What once was a controversy over water versus electrolyte drinks seems to be moving toward a discussion of which electrolyte drink is best. Water alone has not proved to achieve the complete rehydration that athletes need. Fluid replacement is essential to maintain plasma volume necessary for circulation and sweating, and while plain water empties rapidly from your stomach, it tends to dilute plasma concentrations of sodium and stimulate urine output. Water also reduces your feelings of thirst, which is a necessary reminder for you to continue fluid intake. Most experts agree, however, that you should not drink caffeinated or alcoholic beverages before, during, or after exercise. These types of drinks will cause you to become dehydrated. Whatever you choose to drink during exercise, be sure to drink before you start, during your activity, and after you finish.

5. Use the proper equipment for your activity. Your sports equipment should fit you well, be in good working order, and be comfortable. Ill-fitting equipment, such as the wrong size bicycle or hockey skates that are too large, can be a primary cause of sports injuries. Getting good equipment is making an investment in yourself. If your equipment is uncomfortable or broken, you open yourself not only to injury, but also to discouragement. You may not perform as well or have as much fun as you would with reliable equipment, and consequently, you may not choose to participate in that sport again. Although we suggest good equipment, it does not have to be the most expensive, top-of-the-line product you can find. By reading magazines in your chosen sport, visiting professionally staffed stores, and trying out various brands, you should be able to make an educated, cost-effective choice.

Be sure to check out the new lines of sports equipment that are specially sized and designed for women, including bikes, running shoes, ski boots, and weight machines. These products have been a real boon, particularly for smaller women who have a hard time finding men's equipment that will fit them. While we are encouraged by this trend, and hope that it continues, we always urge women to be cautious buyers. Be aware that some women's equipment is still not as well designed as men's. A classic case is the mixte bicycle frame that has a downward sloping top tube rather than a horizontal one (presumably so you could ride with a skirt on). Structurally, mixte frames are not as strong as the men's diamond-shaped frames and have been known to break under pressure. In cases such as these, buy the best equipment available as long as you can find the right fit for yourself.

6. Be consistent with your exercise program. Check the waiting room of any sports medicine clinic on Monday morning, and you're likely to find a good number of achy weekend athletes. Take the woman, for example, who plays tennis every other weekend and then heads for the ski slopes for a week of all-day, every-day activity, and she becomes injured. Even though she is regularly active, her body is not primed for this intensity or type of activity. If she had been doing strengthening exercises, or perhaps bicycling consistently for a few months before the trip, she might have been less prone to injury.

In any sport, the best way to avoid injury is to set up and maintain a program that balances all three aspects of physical conditioning—strength, flexibility, and endurance. An aerobics class that begins with stretching, moves into aerobic movement and strengthening exercises, and ends with stretching again is a good example of a balanced workout.

If you want to maintain fitness, physical activity should become part of your lifestyle for at least a half hour three days a week. Also, you will receive more benefits from your exercise program if you do it every other day, rather than three days in a row.

7. Don't overdo it. This is especially important for women who are beginning an exercise program. Often our enthusiasm will push us to do more than our bodies can manage. For example, it is not realistic to think you can run a marathon three months after starting a running program.

8. Increase the intensity and duration of your physical activity gradually. Adding a little more each time you exercise is a sensible way to reach your fitness goals. If you are making a change in your exercise pattern, incorporate that change slowly. If you decide to add speed intervals to your swimming program, for example, add a few intervals at a time until you reach your desired number of sets. The following day, you may want to take an easy swim, go for a walk, or rest.

9. Rest. Rest is as important to your fitness program as any other aspect. On the days you rest, your muscles recover from the exertion of your previous activity. The more strenuous your physical activity, the greater the need for you to rest. Note that if you participate in more than one sport, it is possible to rest in one sport by doing another. For example, if bicycling is your primary sport, a restful day might be an easy swim at a nearby lake.

10. Pay attention to weather conditions. If you exercise out-of-doors, weather can greatly affect your workouts. For instance, if you are planning a long bicycle ride and find it is pouring and 40 degrees F outside, you may choose to postpone or alter your ride. If you do choose to do the long ride, you will need to dress appropriately and take along a change of clothes in case you get wet. Similarly, if you are planning your weekly running speed workout for noon on a 98 degree F day, you may want to consider postponing it.

11. Listen to your body. Your body will often give you clues when it is worn down or getting injured, but many of us ignore them. Pain, sleeplessness, irritability, fatigue, or slower reflexes may be signs that you are overtraining. Your body is sending you the message to take it easy for a while. If you are becoming fatigued, a day off from your exercise program may be just what you need. Also, think twice about exercising when you are getting sick. Exercise may make you feel better mentally, but it may prolong or aggravate a cold or illness. If you are running a fever, plan on resting.

Adapting to weather includes dressing properly for both temperature and weather conditions. In cold weather, dressing in layers of clothing keeps you warmer than one or two heavy articles. This is because air warmed by your body heat becomes trapped in-between layers of clothing, keeping you warm longer. If it is cold and windy, you will want to include an outer layer of wind-breaking fabric. It is especially important to wear a hat in cold weather, because much of your body heat is lost through the top of your head.

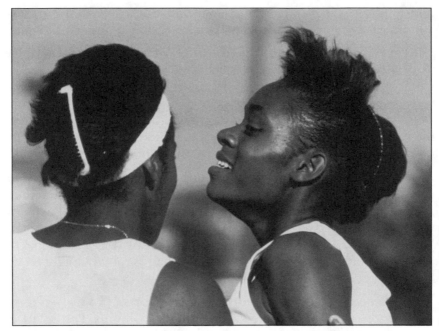

Courtesy of the *Daily Illini*

Overtraining and fatigue may lead to injury. Listen to your body!

On windy days, you may want to think about the prevailing wind direction before you set your course. If you head out into the wind on a run, bike ride, or cross-country ski, the wind will be at your back when you turn around to come home. You will feel a bit warmer, and the wind will gently push you on your way. If you head out with the wind at your back, however, you will find yourself fighting the wind all the way home. Winds also may become stronger and colder in the afternoon, when you are most apt to start tiring. Precipitation is another element you'll learn to respect if you spend much time out-of-doors. Even a warm rain can chill you if you become soaked to the skin. Don't forget to pack a waterproof or water-resistant outer layer if the skies are threatening rain or snow.

Clothes for hot-weather workouts should be light and comfortable. If you tend to perspire a lot, you may want to avoid cotton because it absorbs sweat and becomes heavy and uncomfortable. Instead, you may be better off with clothes made of polypropylene or a similar fiber that wicks moisture away from your body so it can be quickly evaporated into the air. Don't forget the parts of your skin that are exposed; sunscreen is a must if you are out in the sun for long periods of time.

12. Know the signs of impending overuse injury. We all know we're hurt when we have a traumatic injury such as a sprained ankle or a twisted knee, but overuse injuries from exercise can be sneaky. It may be difficult to know if you are really injured or just suffering the common aches, pains, and sore muscles that accompany an active lifestyle.

These are some common signs of an overuse injury:

- Pain. Joint pain or pain when you touch a specific site can be a sign of trouble. Pain lasting hours after a workout or persisting into the following day may indicate impending injury.
- Swelling. Swelling is obvious in some injuries, but in others, the area may just feel swollen without actually changing in size. It may help to compare the size and the sensitivity of that body part with the same part on the other side.
- Reduced range of motion. You may have an overuse injury if you are limited in movement in a muscle or joint when compared with the other side, or if you detect weakness. For instance, if you are favoring a leg because you feel your knee might "go out" on you, you may be overdoing an activity.

13. Know how to treat an overuse injury. Several steps are recommended if you have an overuse injury, or if you suspect that you might be injured:

- Stop doing any activity that causes you pain or that seems to aggravate your injury. You may want to seek medical help if you think the injury is traumatic enough.
- If there is swelling from your injury, you will want to keep it to a minimum.

To reduce swelling just think **R.I.C.E**.

Rest. The only way your injury is really going to heal is by resting.

Ice the injury as soon as possible after the injury occurs. Continue to ice intermittently for the first 20 to 24 hours. Crushed ice, a soft ice pack, or even a bag of frozen peas works best because you can mold it around the injured body part. Note that heat will not reduce swelling; instead, heat actually increases blood flow and swelling. Ice the injured area for 20 to 30 minutes and then remove the ice for 20 to 30 minutes. If you injured a small area, such as your finger, keep the ice on for only 10 to 15 minutes.

Compression. Compress to keep the swelling down; wrap the injured area with an ace bandage. Although you want to limit circulation, be careful not to wrap it so tightly that circulation is completely cut off from that area.

Elevate the injured part of the body as much as possible during the first 24 hours to help keep swelling down.

- You may choose to switch sports for a while until your injury heals. If you do, be sure the activity you substitute doesn't further stress your injury. For example, if you have shin pain from your aerobics class, changing to running will not give your shins a break. Instead, you would want a sport that is non-jarring, such as cycling or swimming.
- You will want to seek medical treatment if the injury is still painful several days later, if swelling persists, if range of motion is severely limited, or if your injury has lasted more than a week or two with rest.

14. Add variety. Having a variety of sports and activities may also help prevent injury. Many overuse injuries occur because we are using the same muscles and joints over and over again and not giving them any chance to recover. By switching to another activity, you give the muscles and joints the recovery they need.

PEAK PERFORMANCE

As you become physically active, it is natural to want to strive to get better and improve your performance. Not all of us are going to become elite athletes, and many may not be interested in competing. However, that does not mean you won't be able to experience the sensation of having a peak performance, just as an elite athlete does. Our research at Melpomene has shown that peak performance can mean many different things to different women. We asked our members what they had to say about peak performances. Are they something that only elite athletes experience? Is a peak performance the same as a "runner's high"? Does it happen only to runners, or could cyclists, swimmers, and golfers experience the same thing? Do peak performances happen only in structured, competitive situations?

Our members responded enthusiastically. Some considered peak performance to be the same as a "peak experience"—a term that was coined by Abraham Maslow, the humanistic psychologist. Maslow believed that a self-actualized person could expect to have peak experiences—moments of highest happiness and fulfillment, characterized by loss of fears, inhibitions, and insecurities. These were moments of total peace and well-being. This definition refers to a subjective emotional state.

Other Melpomene members saw peak performance in terms of objective measures of success, such as winning a race or achieving a "personal best." This view of peak performance is common among many people in sports, especially those in competitive sports. Of

Sandra Bestland: Living Her Dream

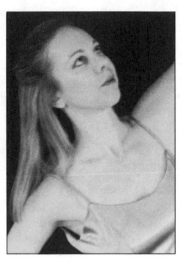

When you watch an Olympic skier turn in a dramatic downhill race, do you wish you had the discipline and strength to learn that sport? When you watch Bonnie Blair on the ice, do you recall the way you felt as a child when you strapped on your skates and felt free and powerful, even graceful?

While fantasizing and recalling are fun, they do little for your physical well-being. To move from the dream to reality takes time, determination, and some-times courage. For **Sandra Bestland**, the motivation to make her dreams come true stemmed from her need to get out of the competitive rat race of corporate life and return to a childhood love: dancing.

"I think the desire to dance had been incubating unconsciously for many years. When I left my twelve-year career as a corporate manager, the first thing I did was sign up for dance classes.

"I had participated in modern dance in college and stayed physically active by practicing yoga, in-line skating around the lakes, and running. In 1987 I even ran the Twin Cities Marathon."

But the next year Sandra decided to get serious about dance. She started dance classes at the Nancy Hauser Dance Studio and worked at her apprenticeship for three years. "Today I spend at least two days a week in the studio just to stay in practice. When I'm rehearsing for a performance at Nancy Hauser, the Walker Art Center, or Hennepin Center for the Arts, I'm at the studio every day.

"Getting re-involved in dance was a gratifying decision for me. At the age I reentered, I wanted people to think that I was good enough to be in productions. My self-esteem soared when my peers confirmed that I was indeed good enough." Today, Sandra dances in at least one production each year with "The Composers," a group of dancers and musicians who collaborate on original performance pieces.

Sandra talks about the role physical activity plays in reducing stress. "As you move you can feel the tension flowing through your body and escaping out your fingers. For me, dancing is also a way to communicate without words. It is a metaphor for life. When I dance, I engage the emotional, physical, intellectual, and spiritual parts of myself."

course, the subjective feeling about which Maslow talks may occur at the same time that the objective record is being broken. What our Melpomene members taught us is that there need not be a medal or a trophy at the end of the race in order to experience a peak performance. All that's really needed is a sense of accomplishment.

For example, one woman wrote, "I ran my first marathon . . . and the emotional and physical high . . . can only compare to childbirth." Another woman recalled that after her first marathon, "I cried I was so happy. Never had I felt such a sense of accomplishment. I had done something totally on my own and succeeded."

Quotes from members participating in many different activities reveal these characteristics. It is also clear that a "peak performance" is a very personal, self-defined accomplishment.

> "When I ran my first 20-mile race . . . I had an overwhelming sense of my body as a finely tuned piece of machinery, and I had control over all the gears. I was able to shift gears for hills and visualized my hips as if the gears were similar to those on my bike. It was an amazing experience to me, and the feeling that I had complete control of my performance turned out to be very relaxing."

> "In 1980 my whole ski season was incredible. Every race was good—I was fast and felt terrific. The last race was great—felt in control and on top of things the whole way—a fantastic experience!"

> "During the finals of the national singles championship in 1971, the background blended together and I was aware of nothing but the shuttlecock. I was totally oblivious to fatigue and pain, and my movements felt smooth and gliding, without conscious effort."

> "In long-distance canoe races I feel very in touch with self and environment—a wonderful sense of mastery and accomplishment."

Peak performance is characterized by relaxation and a sense of power and energy. It has also been described as a feeling of being in control, or an experience of joy and freedom. To strive for that experience through physical activity is a wonderful way to take care of yourself.

SPECIFIC SPORT GUIDELINES

Research has shown that the benefits of exercise are wide-ranging, from stress reduction to protection against illness to personal growth.

Many adult women were not encouraged to be physically active as children, and so sometimes are unsure of how to incorporate exercise into their lifestyles. A few simple strategies, however, can increase the possibility of long-term exercise success. These include selecting the right activity, going slowly, finding an exercise partner, setting goals, and alternating activities. Following simple guidelines for various kinds of sports, such as running or lifting weights, will reduce the possibility of injuries and help make physical activity successful and fun.

We end this chapter with some guidelines for specific physical activities. We have asked experts in each area to list the benefits of the activity and the equipment needed as well as how to get started and how to get better, once you feel that you have built a good foundation. If you are not currently active, we hope you will consider one of these activities or find an activity on your own that you will enjoy. Remember, any activity is better than none at all!

AEROBIC DANCE

Benefits

- Increases aerobic capacity.
- Lowers weight, body fat, and blood pressure.
- Tones muscles.
- Maintains or increases flexibility.

Equipment Tips

While you might think that you must have a bright Lycra outfit to enter the aerobics studio, fashionable clothing is not necessary. All you really need are comfortable clothes in which you can move and a good pair of shoes. Most athletic shoe companies make shoes specifically for aerobics. Look for aerobics shoes that support both lateral and front/back movement and have good shock-absorbing ability.

Getting Started

The motivation for taking an aerobics class should come from you, not from your friends, relatives, or coworkers. The only plan you can realistically stick to is one that you have in your heart.

Be choosy when considering what class(es) you should try. Check with various agencies and facilities to find out what kinds of programs are offered and if their instructors are appropriately certified for the specific classes they're teaching (Aerobic Studio, Water Aerobic Resistance, etc.). Ask if you can "test-drive" a class before signing up.

The class should match your present fitness level and include the following elements: a warm-up, cardiovascular training, flexibility, muscle toning components, and a cool-down. If you are completely fatigued following the trial class, it may be too advanced for you. You should feel invigorated, not spent. For any activity, a good rule of thumb for exercise intensity is that you should be able to converse while exercising.

Getting Better

For a higher-intensity aerobic workout you may want to take a more advanced class. You can also increase your workout by increasing your rhythm (speed) in the class you are currently taking. Greater flexibility can be achieved through full extension of your arms and legs during a class at any level.

You may also want to target your weakest area for strengthening. For example, you may be able to make it through your aerobics class feeling strong and energized. However, during the stretching portions, you find that you can barely do the stretches that the instructor is demonstrating. In such a case, you might want to stretch outside of class daily to increase your overall flexibility.

Martha Stoll Albertson
Exercise Physiologist at The Marsh, a Center
for Health and Balance, Minnetonka, Minnesota

WEIGHT LIFTING

Benefits

- Increases strength.
- Tones muscles.
- Builds stronger bones.

Equipment Tips

Different kinds of weight equipment are used in weight training to accomplish various results.

Weight machines. Machines are used to work specific muscle groups. The two most common types of weight training machines are pivot machines and cam machines. Both are designed to allow a specific muscle group to complete a full range of motion. Many women find that if they use weight machines regularly, it is important to find a facility that has women's equipment. This equipment tends to be smaller and easier for women to use.

Free weights. Free weights refers to lifting weights without the aid of a machine. The weights are called "free" because the equipment does not restrict joint movement. It is especially important to make sure that you maintain proper form with free weights, since there is no machine to "guide" you through the motions. Injuries are likely when you don't use correct loading, lifting, and spotting techniques.

Getting Started

How many women have ventured into a weight room, only to discover it full of thick-necked, muscle-bound men named Biff? Fortunately, not all weight rooms are like that. As more and more women begin lifting weights, the weight room is changing. Ask friends or make inquiries to help you find a facility that welcomes and encourages women.

Although weight training offers many benefits, it also is one form of exercise in which you can injure yourself without the proper techniques. Many books and even magazines discuss weight training techniques and exercises, and many health clubs have a personal trainer you can use to help set up a weight training program.

To avoid injury, it's important to warm up before you begin lifting. A warm-up should consist of 5 minutes of aerobic activity such as jogging or jumping rope to prepare your muscles. After a warm-up, it's a good idea to stretch before you begin lifting. When lifting free weights, particularly the heavier weights, it is important to have a partner to spot you and who is able to assist you if you need help.

Before beginning a workout program it's good to have a goal in mind—are you lifting to increase strength, keep muscle tone, or a bit of both? The lighter the resistance along with more repetitions, the more endurance and muscle tone you will maintain. During endurance training it's suggested to use two sets of 10 reps for each lift. Between sets you should allow a 1-1/2-to-2-minute rest. A strength program, on the other hand, consists of fewer reps with heavy resistance.

Repetitions (Reps): The number of times a weight is continuously lifted.

Set: Each group of repetitions.

For example: If you do eight arm curls and rest and eight more arm curls before moving on to another exercise, you will have completed two sets of eight reps on arm curls.

Adapted from N. Mood, 1991, *Sports and Recreational Activities*, 10th ed. (St. Louis: Mosby-Year Book).

Once you have started a weight lifting program you may want to keep a journal. This allows you to look back and see the progress you've made. Be sure to include the exercises you've done, the number of sets and reps, and the amount of weight.

Try not to work one muscle group without working the opposing group. For example: It's not good to focus on biceps without working your triceps. Start with the larger muscle groups, moving to the smaller, alternating between upper and lower body.

Lifting three times a week is ideal, since it gives you a day to rest in-between workouts and allows your muscles to rebuild themselves.

Proper breathing while you are lifting is also important. Rather than holding your breath, you should inhale during the lowering phase of the lift and exhale during the working phase.

To add variety to your weight lifting workouts you might want to add circuit training or isometric exercises to your routine. Circuit training involves aerobic (using oxygen) as well as anaerobic (not using oxygen) work capacities. A circuit workout consists of 8-12 stations. Ten to 12 reps should be completed at each station, or, even better, complete as many reps as you can in a certain time limit (30-45 seconds). You should rotate time lifting with jogging in place or bike riding to keep your heart rate up.

Isometric exercising involves working against resistance that cannot be moved. For this, you may wish to involve a partner. For example, one person may hold the end of a towel and lift while, at the same time, the partner is pushing downward on the towel, creating resistance.

Getting Better

The best way to build maximum strength is the 8-5-2 program. This means that the first set consists of eight repetitions (reps), the second set five reps, and the third set two reps. With each set, you will increase the weight 10 percent—from 70 percent to 80 percent to 90 percent of the maximum weight you can lift. You can find the maximum weight you can lift for each exercise through trial and error.

The first time in the weight room it's best to start out with lighter weights. Rather than lifting 100 percent of your maximum, 90 percent is the most you should lift to avoid injury. For example, if 75 pounds is your maximum, you would lift eight reps at 50 pounds (approximately 70 percent), five reps at 60 pounds (80 percent), and two reps at 70 pounds (90 percent). After you can lift three reps at 90 percent, you should move your maximum weight up by 5 pounds and from there figure out what 70, 80, and 90 percent of that weight is.

Sharon Saydah
Personal Fitness Trainer

CROSS-COUNTRY SKIING

Benefits

- Excellent aerobic conditioning exercise.
- Uses most of your major muscle groups.
- Provides a seasonal sport alternative.

Equipment Tips

Touring cross-country skis. These versatile skis are intended for diagonal-stride (Nordic) traditional skiing. They come in either waxable or waxless styles. The difference is that waxless skis can be used without having to prepare the bottom surfaces with waxes. In place of wax, plastic "fish scales" on the bottom of the ski grip the snow in almost any weather condition. The disadvantage is that waxless skis are not very fast. If you plan to ski often during a winter, you will probably want to consider the faster waxable skis, even though you will have to "wax up" before you head out. Contrary to popular belief, the waxing process does not have to be complex, and it will give you a quicker, more responsive glide than you can get with most waxless skis.

Skating skis. Skating skis are designed specifically for a technique called skating, which has become popular in the last 10 years. Skating involves more of a herring-bone stride than Nordic skiing. The skating ski is stiffer, has a built-up sidewall, and is shorter. It is helpful to have all skis professionally fitted to your particular height, weight, and type of skiing.

Boots. Boots for skating skis have a high top to provide more ankle support. When buying boots, a beginning skier can generally start at the bottom end of the price range and expect equipment to last for many years.

Poles. Poles also vary in price and strength depending on use. Skating poles are longer, stronger, and more expensive. Again, it is important to have ski poles that fit your height and anticipated use.

Fanny pack. Many people wear a small fanny pack when skiing that holds some snacks, lip protection, sun protection, and water. Cross-country skiing any distance will usually cause you to sweat, so it is a good idea to drink before you start as well as during your ski to prevent dehydration.

Getting Started

Dressing correctly is a key to comfort. An ideal temperature range for cross-country skiing is 10 to 22 degrees F, but since most skiers will find only a few ideal days per season, it is important to know how to dress for any weather. For the most part, people tend to overdress. In addition to considering factors such as wind, snow, sun, and clouds, your pace and intensity of skiing will also influence how much you should wear. Remember that you will be using your whole body and will most likely warm up quickly. Wearing layered clothing that you can remove and put in your pack is an excellent idea. If the weather is below 10 degrees, it is smart to wear some sort of polypropylene product which will wick water away from your body and keep you warmer. Avoid wearing clothes made of cotton, because they become heavy when they get wet and will feel clammy and cold when you stop exercising. Remember to wear a hat in colder weather and to have a face mask if the temperature is below zero. Warm gloves or mittens are another important requirement. Though most ski boots now are lined with an insulating inner liner, wool socks are a must. Lightweight polypropylene socks to be worn under the wool socks are a good idea for particularly cold weather. It is also possible to buy a bootie which goes over your boot and adds further warmth for particularly cold days.

Consider taking lessons. While diagonal-stride skiing is a fairly easy technique to master, we recommend that you rent skis for your first try, and get a lesson at the same time. The hints provided by a good instructor will make skiing far more pleasurable. Most people who decide to try the skating method also take at least one lesson. While it may look easy, a few suggestions and technique tips make it much more efficient and fun.

Choose an appropriate place to ski. Golf courses and parks are a good place to start skiing, and an increasing number of parks now provide skis for rental at a reasonable rate. Almost all ski areas have well-marked trails which also let you know degree of difficulty. An "easiest" trail may vary in difficulty among geographical regions of the United States, so it is smart to ask about unfamiliar trails before you start. Most trail systems will also have the length of the trail marked so that you can judge how long you will be out.

Getting Better

Try some intermediate and, eventually, some advanced trails. Challenge yourself, however, don't get into situations that will be frustratingly difficult or even dangerous. Ask someone at the warming hut or visitor center to describe the trail conditions before you head out.

Try racing. Cross-country ski racing is gaining in popularity across the U.S. Look for races in your local paper, or see if there is a ski club in your area. Many races have 5- or 10-year age divisions. Distances for cross-country races vary greatly, from 5K to the famous Birkebinder held every year in Hayward, Wisconsin, which is 55K in length. Terrain and weather conditions mean it is much harder to predict your time on a course, but competitive women in their twenties are able to ski a 10K in 29 minutes; excellent times for women in their forties are in the 35-minute range.

Judy Mahle Lutter
Melpomene Cofounder and President

BICYCLING

Benefits

- Increases aerobic capacity.
- Low impact.
- Can be used as a form of transportation.

Equipment Tips

Choose the kind of bike that is best for you. Three main types of bicycles dominate the market: mountain bikes, hybrids (city bikes), and road (racing or touring) bikes. Questions to consider before buying a bike include: What type of riding do I plan on doing? Am I interested in mountain biking—tackling dirt trails and other obstacles? Am I planning to ride mostly on paved bike paths? Will I participate in road races? Are there certain features I am looking for in a bicycle? Read a biking magazine or talk to a friend who bikes so that you are prepared when shopping for a bike.

Adjust your seat so you are neither too high nor too low. Even an inch can put undo stress on your knees. To find the proper height for your seat, have a friend stand behind you and watch as you pedal. The seat should be low enough so that your hips don't shift from side to side. When your leg is at the bottom of the stroke, it should be slightly bent at the knee. Another way to measure height is to put your heel on the pedal and fully extend your leg. In this position, your leg should be almost straight, with little bend in the knee.

Make sure you are not too stretched out or cramped on your bike. It's natural for your shoulders and neck to hurt on the first few rides of the season, but if the pain continues, visit your local bike shop. Ask them about changing the length of your handlebar stem, moving your seat back or forth, or tilting the seat up a bit.

If you are saddle sore, try wearing a good pair of cycling shorts with a real chamois or synthetic chamois padding. Look for a pair of cycling shorts that do not have a seam in the middle of the crotch area. It might seem unimportant at first, but after a long ride you'll notice the difference. Bike shorts are meant to be worn without underwear. If this doesn't help, look into buying a new seat. Seats come in a variety of widths, and some are now made with a gel material that cushions the pressure points upon which you sit.

Always wear a helmet. Even the best riders are victims of motorists' mistakes.

Wear well-padded cycling gloves, and change hand positions frequently.

Getting Started

1. Keep your cadence high (60-100 revolutions per minute) to avoid overtiring your legs, and bend your elbows slightly to decrease stress on your joints.
2. Ride three to five days a week, if possible. Ride a comfortable distance at a lively pace. For a harder workout, do either the speed, power, or hill workout below.
3. Find a group of people who are at your level or a little better to ride with. Each week, increase the speed and distance of your ride.

Getting Better

Here are some sample workouts to help you improve various aspects of your biking performance.

Speed. Sprint 200 yards at top speed, recover completely, and repeat until you can no longer maintain your form or speed.

Endurance. Do one long ride each week, increasing the length weekly. Keep the pace snappy. A long, slow ride does not result in improvement.

Power. In a high gear, stand up and ride for several minutes. Recover to a heart rate of 70 percent of maximum (220 minus your age), and do this five or six times. Or do decreasing intervals of two minutes, one and a half minutes, one minute, and a half minute, letting your heart recover to 70 percent between each one.

Hill climbing. Ride a few hills each time you go out. Find a two- or three-minute hill, and give it your all five or six times, pacing yourself to keep a steady momentum all the way to the top. Shift into a low gear at the bottom of the hill and "spin" at a high cadence until you meet the resistance of the hill.

Form. Have another cyclist check to see that your back is flat when you are in a crouched position. Try to pedal with only one leg in order to find and eliminate the dead spots in your revolution.

Megan Webster
United States Cycling Federation (USCF) Racer

SWIMMING

Benefits

- Excellent way to develop cardiorespiratory fitness.
- Uses most of the major muscle groups.
- Is continuous in nature and can be done at a moderate pace.
- Injuries are rare because swimming puts less stress on joints and muscles than weight-bearing exercises do (water buoys you up!).
- Can be enjoyed throughout one's lifetime, leisurely or competitively.
- Can be done individually, with a friend, or with a group.

Equipment Tips

Swimsuit. Nylon adds durability to a suit, and Lycra adds comfort. Both are important if you intend to swim regularly.

Goggles. If you haven't used goggles before, we recommend that you take time to find some that are comfortable and that fit your face. Goggles improve vision and reduce eye irritation. They allow you to see where you are going, monitor your arm action, and generally make swimming more enjoyable. Goggles come in a variety of colors and shapes to fit anyone, but they require a period of adjustment. After about a week of making minor adjustments to the nose piece and the sides, you'll find they'll fit you like a glove and you won't want to swim without them. If fogging is a problem, try using a defogging solution, or buy non-fogging goggles.

Getting Started

1. Consider taking lessons. With basic training, anyone can learn to swim or learn to swim more efficiently. Check with your local community swimming program, the YMCA/YWCA, local high schools or colleges, or a nearby health club. You can usually choose either group instruction or private lessons.
2. Find a pool that has scheduled times for adults to swim laps and that uses lane lines (on the bottom of the pool) to separate the swimmers into groups.
3. Check with the lifeguard regarding lane pace at your pool. Most lap swim programs have slow lanes, medium pace, and fast lanes. Also check the circle pattern which establishes the direction of travel around the black lines on the bottom of the pool. You will swim up one side of the line and down the other, going

clockwise or counterclockwise depending on the rules at your pool. When you are just beginning, choose the slow lanes, and stop at each end of the pool, pausing at the corner to let other swimmers pass by.

4. Start slowly, and build into a swimming program. You will be amazed at how quickly you can increase your water endurance each time. Keep your swimming strokes long and stretched, and enjoy your individual progress. Rushing yourself at first will only lead to muscle soreness because your body is not yet used to the exercise.

Getting Better

Challenge yourself to improve in the three basic parts of training known by the abbreviation F.I.T.

Frequency
- One day a week is better than none.
- Three times a week is recommended for a training effect.

Intensity
- Begin at your level, and go slowly.
- As your skill improves, monitor your heart rate by counting the pulses for 15 seconds, then multiply by 4. If you want to improve your fitness level, you should be swimming fast enough to get your heart rate up to at least 120.

Time
- You can begin with as little as 10 minutes.
- To make significant improvements you should swim for 30-60 minutes.

Add variety to your workouts. Try spicing up your distance (continuous) workouts with interval swimming (swimming and resting patterns), kicking with sideboards, pulling with pull-buoys, and/or a combination of these. Motivation and innovation within your program are limited only by your own creativeness.

Try working out with a group. For swimmers 19 and older, Masters Swimming is offered at pools and health clubs throughout the nation, with competition available in 5-year age groups. Whatever your level of swimming, remember to swim for the fun of it.

Sharon Simpson
Coach and Masters Swimmer

WATER EXERCISE

Benefits

- Increases aerobic capacity.
- Tones muscles.
- Maintains or increases flexibility.
- Low or no impact—ideal for older or larger exercisers, and for people with musculoskeletal injuries or chronic illness such as arthritis.

Equipment Tips

A comfortable bathing suit is the only necessity for water exercise. Water shoes are recommended, as they protect your feet if you are walking on the floor of a pool. Water shoes also prevent slipping and help you to maintain a stationary position as you exercise.

Optional equipment (depending on the class you are taking) includes milk jugs filled with air to increase resistance or equipment to make you buoyant for zero impact while you exercise.

Getting Started

Water exercise is not just aerobics in the pool. The properties of water, such as buoyancy, resistance, temperature, and depth, need to be taken into consideration when designing an exercise program. Therefore, be sure to inquire about the instructor's certification in water exercise, training, and experience.

Try a class to see if you like it. Don't expect to feel the same exertion level as you would in a studio aerobics class. However, the cardiovascular and resistance benefits will be similar to a land-based program.

Getting Better

Move on to a more advanced class when what was once hard is no longer difficult. As with a land-based aerobics class, you can make your workout harder in the pool by increasing your rhythm, and you can increase flexibility through full limb extension. One word of caution: It may "feel" easier to extend your arms and legs because you are in the water, but to avoid injury, don't stretch beyond what is comfortable.

Martha Stoll Albertson
Exercise Physiologist at The Marsh, a Center for Health and Balance, Minnetonka, Minnesota

WALKING

Benefits

- Increases cardiovascular capacity.
- Weight-bearing exercise, helps prevent osteoporosis.
- Tones muscles.
- Can be done anywhere!

Equipment Tips

The only equipment you need to begin walking for fitness is a good pair of shoes and comfortable clothes. Walking shoes should be light-weight but durable and should not feel big and clunky on your feet.

Getting Started

Walking is one of the easiest ways for most people to begin an exercise program. It's easily incorporated into your day-to-day activities. Some women have found that just parking farther away from the office is a good way for them to begin walking more regularly. Others find walking a great way to spend time talking to others.

If you are not used to walking for long periods of time or great distances, begin with setting reasonable goals. It might be that you begin by saying, "I'm going to walk 10 minutes tonight," or "I'm going to walk around the block two times." By starting slowly you can build up to a comfortable rate and will be less likely to become discouraged. Also, walking is a great activity to do with a friend. Having someone to talk to will make the time go faster and help keep you motivated.

Getting Better

To get the most out of your walk you should aim for a 12-minute mile. Bend your arms at a 90-degree angle, and concentrate on moving them faster. By moving your arms faster you'll begin to move your feet faster, too. Always remember to keep a comfortable stride. If you feel as if you are about to fall forward, you are moving too fast. Also remember to keep your back straight: Leaning too far forward or backward can cause injuries and prevent you from gaining the most from your walk. To keep your back straight, do not look down at your feet. Instead, find a point directly ahead at eye level, and focus on it while you walk.

Sharon Saydah
Personal Fitness Trainer

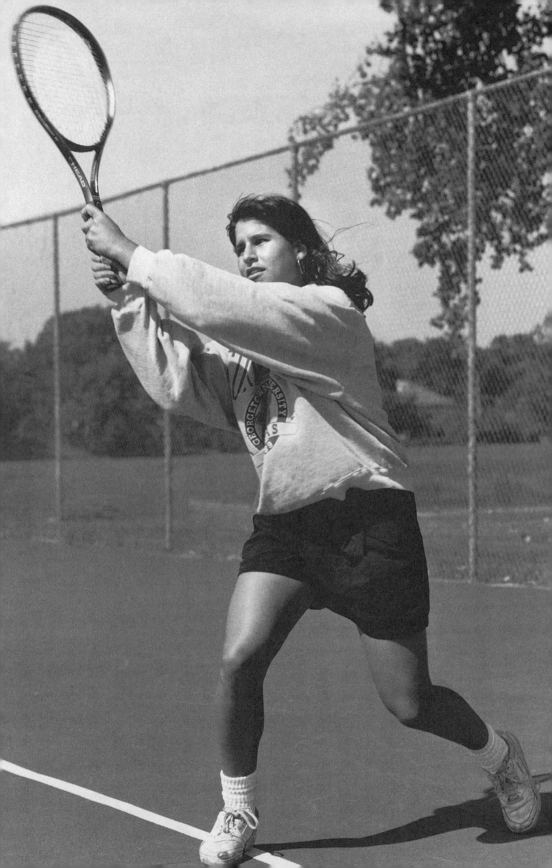

Menstrual Fact and Fiction

Danielle started regular physical activity about 5 years ago. During the warm weather, she plays tennis nearly every day, and in the winter she swims. Danielle noticed that her menstrual periods changed once she became physically active. Cramps were fewer, and the flow seemed lighter. Although these changes were inconsequential, Danielle wondered if they were related to her exercise program.

Cynthia began running 7 years ago. She became serious about the sport when she discovered that she had talent as a runner. Cynthia's training program often includes mileage of 40 to 50 miles per week. As a result of diet change and the high mileage, she has lost about 10 pounds. Cynthia stopped having menstrual periods 3 years ago and is concerned about her health. She wonders if the absence of periods is unhealthy and if she will ever be able to have children.

WHAT IS NORMAL?

Most women have concerns from time to time about their menstrual cycles and reproductive health. Certainly when there is some notice-able change in our bodies, we tend to wonder if we are "normal." When it comes to menstrual functioning, the term normal defies definition and often leaves doctors and researchers baffled. Usually, the average is considered the norm, and if a woman fluctuates far enough away from this average, she may be considered "not normal." We must keep in mind, however, that averages can't describe every case, and what is "not normal" for most women may be perfectly healthy for you.

Most women experience menstrual cycles that are anywhere from 20 to 36 days in length, with an average of 28 days. Usually these cycles are ovulatory, which means that an egg is released about midway through the cycle (about 14 days before bleeding starts). Not every menstrual cycle is ovulatory, however. Occasionally, you may have an anovulatory cycle—one in which an egg is not released.

Hormones of various kinds have major roles in the menstrual cycle. Two of the most prominent are estrogen and progesterone. Estrogen is the key player from day 1 (when bleeding starts) through day 14 of your cycle. Throughout this follicular phase, estrogen is rising and the uterine lining or endometrium is building up, preparing for ovulation and possible pregnancy. Estrogen levels peak just before ovulation, then drop dramatically.

As estrogen is starting to rise during the first week of the cycle, another hormone, called follicle stimulating hormone (FSH), is re-leased by the pituitary gland. FSH, which causes the growth and maturation of ovarian follicles in preparation for ovulation, is at a slightly elevated level during the first week and then drops off again until about day 14. When ovulation is about to occur, FSH and a fourth hormone called luteinizing hormone (LH) both rise to peak levels which cause a now mature follicle to release the egg.

For the next 2 weeks of the cycle, or the luteal phase, there is a rise in progesterone, a hormone that "ripens" the endometrium. As progesterone decreases toward the end of this luteal phase, and if no pregnancy has occurred, bleeding will begin, and the menstrual flow will last about 4 to 7 days. The figure on the next page illustrates hormonal levels during the menstrual cycle.

Again, not all women fit this average profile, and this does not mean that their health is in danger. Rather, they may be experiencing wider fluctuations within what is still considered the normal and healthy range. For example, while the interval between ovulation and

Changes in Hormone Levels During the Menstrual Cycle

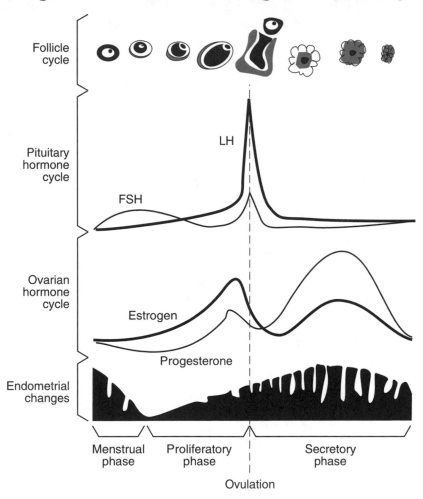

Follicle
cycle

Pituitary
hormone
cycle

LH

FSH

Ovarian
hormone
cycle

Estrogen

Progesterone

Endometrial
changes

Menstrual
phase

Proliferatory
phase

Secretory
phase

Ovulation

Reprinted, by permission, from Boston Women's Health Book Collective, 1992, *The New Our Bodies, Ourselves*. (New York: Touchstone Books), 256.

menstrual flow is usually constant at 14 days, the preovulatory period from menstruation to ovulation may vary from 7 days to 30 days or more in some women, which explains why menstrual cycles sometimes vary in length. A number of factors can affect menstrual timing and flow, including diet, stress, weight loss, and physical activity. In this chapter, we will look at how your exercise program may or may not impact your menstrual cycle, and what changes you might expect over time. We've included a brief glossary on page 142 to help you with the terminology.

Glossary

Amenorrhea—The absence of menstruation. A woman who has primary amenorrhea has never menstruated; she has not yet reached menarche. A woman who has secondary amenorrhea has reached menarche but has stopped menstruating since then.

Anovulatory cycle—A cycle in which no egg is released from the ovaries.

Bone mass—The total amount of bone in the skeleton.

Corpus luteum—Latin for "yellow body." The corpus luteum is formed by the thecal and granulosa cells which are left behind after the egg is released from the ovaries. The corpus luteum produces estrogen and progesterone for 14 days and then degenerates if no pregnancy occurs. If pregnancy does occur, the corpus luteum produces hormones for 4 months until the placenta takes over hormone production.

Dysmenorrhea—Painful menstruation.

Estrogen—The hormone responsible for the development and maintenance of female sex characteristics and reproductive function in women. Estrogens are produced by the ovaries. Estrogen is responsible for the first half of the menstrual cycle. Among other effects, estrogens thicken the endometrium, promote conception, enhance bone development/formation, and cause low-density lipoproteins to decrease. (See also progesterone.)

Eumenorrhea—Regularly occurring periods.

Follicular phase—The preovulatory phase of the menstrual cycle when follicles are stimulated by hormones so that one will eventually mature into an egg. (See also luteal phase.)

Hyperprolactinemia—Elevated levels of the hormone prolactin. Prolactin is the hormone responsible for milk production which, when elevated, can play a role in

(cont.)

Glossary (cont.)

menstrual irregularities (e.g., nursing women may not have their periods for some time).

Hypothalamus—A gland in the lower part of the brain that manufactures some hormones and controls the release of other hormones from the pituitary gland. Significantly, the hypothalamus controls the release of follicle stimulating hormone (which causes a follicle to develop into a mature ovum) and luteinizing hormone (which causes the formation of the corpus luteum).

Hypothyroidism—A condition of low thyroid function which may affect menstrual function.

Luteal phase—The postovulatory phase of the menstrual cycle in which the corpus luteum produces hormones. The endometrium is prepared for implantation under the influence of the hormones produced by the corpus luteum. (See also follicular phase.)

Menarche—The first occurrence of menstruation.

Oligomenorrhea—Irregularly occurring menstruation.

Osteoporosis—A reduction in overall bone mass characterized by increased porosity and thinning of the bones. Osteoporosis is directly related to loss of estrogen and also to interactions among genetic, nutritional, and environmental factors. Bone mass generally reaches its peak when a woman is in her thirties and gradually declines thereafter, accelerating after menopause. Bones weakened by osteoporosis are more susceptible to fracture.

Progesterone—A hormone produced by the ovary during the second half of the menstrual cycle. Progesterone acts to prepare the uterus for pregnancy. (See also estrogen.)

*Thanks to Michonne Bertrand for providing this glossary.

MENSTRUAL DISCOMFORT

"I often need to curtail my physical activity during the first days of my period due to increased flow and cramping."

"Throughout high school and the first 2 years of college, I was almost bedridden with severe cramping, nausea, vomiting, and heavy bleeding due to my period. I missed school and was on medication."

"I notice my cramping more when I'm running or swimming. It seems more intense."

A common menstrual complaint is dysmenorrhea, characterized by lower abdominal cramps, which may be accompanied by headache, backache, fatigue, breast soreness, and/or weight gain during the menstrual cycle. Researchers in the 1930s were among the first to recognize dysmenorrhea as physical rather than psychological in origin. In the past, researchers linked such factors as bad posture, "faulty living habits," and the lack of abdominal strength to the occurrence of dysmenorrhea.

Myths surrounding the menstrual period are evident in the following quote from the book *Wife and Mother, or Information for Every Woman,* published in 1888, which states:

During "the monthly periods," violent exercise is injurious; iced drinks and acid beverages are improper; and bathing in the sea, and bathing the feet in cold water, and cold baths, are dangerous; indeed, at such times as these, no risks should be run, and no experiments should, for one moment, be permitted, otherwise serious consequences will, in all probability, ensue. "The monthly periods" are times not to be trifled with, or woe betide the unfortunate trifler! . . . The pale, colorless complexion, helpless, listless, and almost lifeless young ladies, that are so constantly seen in society, usually owe their miserable state of health either to absent, to deficient, or to profuse menstruation. Their breathing is short—they are soon "out of breath"; if they attempt to take exercise—to walk, for instance, either up stairs, or up a hill, or even for half a mile on level ground, their breath is nearly exhausted—they pant as though they had been running quickly. They are ready, after the slightest exertion or fatigue, and after the least worry or excitement, to feel faint, and sometimes even to actually swoon away.

Effects of Physical Activity

Remember your high school gym teacher telling you that physical activity is the best way to alleviate menstrual discomfort? Research is showing that this belief is not necessarily true; the relationship between menstrual symptoms and physical activity is more complex than we once thought.

It has been only in the past 25 years that researchers have looked at athletic training and its impact on the menstrual cycle. In a 1975 study of 1,435 students, Dr. Allan J. Ryan, editor-in-chief of *The Physician and Sportsmedicine*, concluded that there is little correlation between the severity of dysmenorrhea and levels of physical activity. Further, a study of Olympic athletes in the 1976 Montreal games found that although almost 60 percent of the women reported some change in their menstrual patterns due to intense physical activity, only 12 percent of the women noted a lessening of abdominal cramps. For 6 percent of the women, cramping reportedly increased as a result of their activity.

In 1984, we sent a questionnaire to all Melpomene members to gather information on their health and lifestyle, and to learn something about their menstrual patterns. The 420 women who answered the questionnaire experienced a wide variety of menstrual symptoms. The most frequently reported symptoms were monthly weight gain, abdominal cramps, irritability, and change in appetite. The women in this study who were sedentary reported cramping, fluctuations in appetite, and mood swings with the same frequency as those women who were active.

More recently, however, researchers Inza Fort, Ro Di Brezzo, and Janet Forbess at the University of Arkansas found that women who exercise on a regular basis report fewer symptoms and decreased menstrual discomfort compared with women who are infrequent exercisers. The 960 participants in this 1990 study were members over the age of 30 of the National Association of Girls and Women in Sport (NAGWS). Participants responded to a questionnaire requesting information about their menstrual cycle. When respondents were broken down into groups according to their level of physical activity, the researchers found that women in the more active groups reported pain and cramping, bloating, and breast tenderness less often than women in groups described as recreational and inactive. However, about half of the women in the most active groups did report experiencing these symptoms at least some of the time.

The benefits of an active lifestyle on the menstrual cycle are mixed. Physical activity, though it may cause lighter or more infrequent periods, will not necessarily "cure" common menstrual symptoms such as cramping, backache, bloating, or breast tenderness. The most notice-able effect of physical activity is more often in menstrual patterns, rather than in the lessening of menstrual discomforts. There are, thank-fully, other treatment options for women who suffer from painful menstrual periods. Athletic women, their coaches, and their physicians should be aware of them.

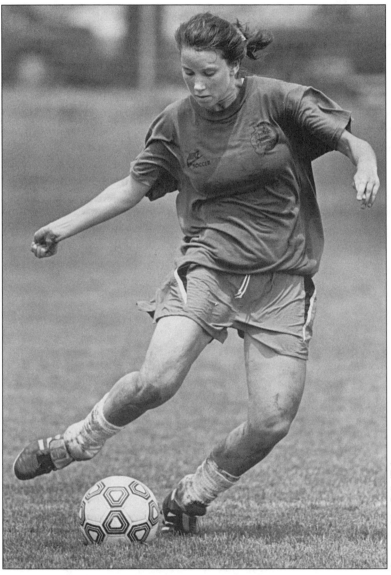

Courtesy of the *Daily Illini*

The benefits of an active lifestyle on the menstrual cycle are mixed.

When to Seek Help

For most women, home remedies or over-the-counter drugs are enough to alleviate menstrual discomfort and cramping. If, however, these methods are not working for you, your next step is to talk with a health-care provider. Your gynecologist is best qualified to treat menstrual cycle discomfort, but it will be important for you to discuss all options with him or her before you undertake any treatment.

Relieving Menstrual Discomfort

Among the natural ways to alleviate discomfort, relaxation techniques and diet changes are often suggested in concert with exercise. Some dietary changes recommended by health-care providers might include eating a balanced diet rich in whole grains, fruits, and vegetables, or adding calcium, either through dietary sources or by taking a daily calcium magnesium supplement. There are also several nonprescription remedies on the market, some producing only pain relief, while others add a diuretic to lessen water retention. Although these remedies alleviate symptoms in some women, they are not effective for all women or women with severe symptoms.

For many years, physicians have routinely prescribed narcotics such as codeine or Percodan to relieve cramping and other menstrual symptoms. While these do a great job of combating pain, they also produce troublesome side effects such as sleepiness, light-headedness, and even nausea. For many women, taking narcotic pain killers is just a way of trading one level of dysfunction for another.

Nonsteroidal anti-inflammatory drugs (NSAIDS) entered the scene in 1984, when ibuprofen became available over-the-counter. Previously available by prescription only, ibuprofen brings many women relief with minimal side effects. In 1994, naproxen sodium also became available without a prescription. These drugs work to inhibit prostaglandins—the substances in your body that cause your uterus, intestines, and other smooth muscles to contract. These contractions produce painful cramps as they squeeze blood from your uterine muscle. Rising levels of prostaglandins are also responsible for the intestinal cramping and diarrhea that many women experience along with menstrual cramps. Prostaglandin-inhibiting drugs block prostaglandin production and activity in the body. These drugs work best if you take them as soon as your flow begins, before your prostaglandin levels are high enough to produce painful cramps. NSAIDS are often less irritating to the

Robyn Hanscom: Running Healthy Now

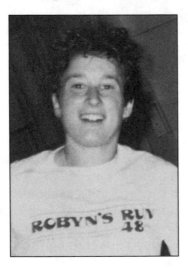

Robyn Hanscom ran her first marathon in 1980 at the age of 29. In March of 1981, she ran a 50-mile race, and in May a 100-kilometer race. During the 7 years beginning in 1980, Robyn averaged running 80 miles each week, and competed in five 24-hour races, two 48-hour races, five 100-kilometer races, twenty 26.2-mile marathons, and four 50-mile ultramarathons.

During these 7 years, Robyn did not have a menstrual period. "Losing my period seemed to coincide with the running. I also went off the pill and got an IUD," Robyn explains. "I was worried about getting an IUD because of the possibility of heavier flow, but I was sick of the pill and the possible side-effects. At first I was concerned about not having my period. But I also felt great and was really into the running. And I sure didn't miss seven years of not buying tampons! "

Robyn saw more than one doctor about her lack of menstrual cycles. "They did all kinds of tests, pituitary x-rays, and blood work, but in the end they decided that it was OK, it must be just from the running. I changed gynecologists during that time, too. My first one was really worried. He thought I should be having children."

Robyn admits that during these years she had an eating disorder. "I had a kind of bulimia, except that I purged by running, not vomiting. I would binge then go run 20 miles the next day."

Robyn was a participant in Melpomene's study of athletic amenorrhea. Through tests associated with the study, she discovered she had a low functioning thyroid, which can affect the menstrual cycle.

"Through the Melpomene study, I was referred to a physician who was more sympathetic and who understood the role of exercise. The doctor thought that the risk of low bone density plus the fact that I was thinking about becoming pregnant meant that we should try to get my cycle back. First she gave me a dose of Clomid. That didn't work, so then she gave me a double dose. There was some spotting but nothing regular. I don't remember having a true cycle, even when I conceived."

Robyn's two children are now six and four. Of her pregnancies, Robyn says, "Physically, they were great. With both kids, I wore a supportive belt I found at a maternity store, and I ran until the very end of my pregnancy. I kept at 20 miles a week until the day before I delivered."

Today Robyn runs regularly, about 20 to 30 miles a week. "I'm still in my running club. I ran with them yesterday after work. Running is very social for me." Of her ultramarathoning days and her eating disorder, Robyn explains, "At that time, I ate and ran partly to escape from my feelings. Now I can feel things, and my running has never felt better."

gastrointestinal tract than aspirin. However, as with any drug, there are side effects, and some people are advised not to take them. This includes women with aspirin-induced asthma or gastrointestinal irritation (e.g., peptic ulcer) and anyone who is sensitive to the particular kind of drug prescribed.

Some health-care providers suggest oral contraceptives, or birth control pills, as a way to relieve severe symptoms. The hormones in oral contraceptives may decrease cramping in several ways. First, they prevent ovulation, and cycles in which no egg is released are usually free from cramping. They also thin the uterine lining and lessen the blood flow, so that uterine contractions are reduced. Finally, oral contraceptives probably quiet menstrual cramping by reducing the amount of prostaglandin precursors (substances that have the potential to become prostaglandins) in the endometrium. Though they are known to be effective for some women, oral contraceptives should be used only when other medical means have been exhausted. Before you decide to go on the pill, you'll want to discuss the risks with your doctor, especially if you are over 35, are a smoker, or are concerned with sports performance. (See contraception discussion on page 172.)

While there is no perfect method for relieving menstrual discomfort, symptoms are no longer being ignored or written off as psychological. Menstrual symptoms are recognized as very real and are receiving well-deserved attention from the medical and scientific community. Another set of changes that affects your menstrual patterns may not be as easy to detect as the symptoms we just discussed. Nevertheless, they can have significant implications for your health. The following section reviews these major changes, their possible connection to exercise, and the current view of treatment.

LATE ONSET OF MENSTRUATION

"Being age 19-1/2 and never having had a period concerned me."

"As early as high school, I consulted a gynecologist about not having my period, but the message was, 'Don't worry; you're just late!'"

A girl's body begins to change noticeably even before she has her first period. She experiences a growth spurt, her breasts develop, her pubic and underarm hair grows, and her body becomes more rounded in places where fat is deposited. Her first period usually comes after some or all of these changes, but it may not become regular or ovulatory for 2 years or longer.

In the United States and western Europe, the typical age of menarche (onset of menstruation) is now 12-1/2, which is somewhat younger than it was 20 years ago. Experts speculate that this drop in menarche age may be due to improved living conditions, better nutrition, or better health care. It may be that children are reaching their full size sooner, achieving a greater weight for their height, or becoming fit and capable of childbearing at a younger age.

In this era of relatively young menarche, it's natural for a girl to become concerned if her first period seems to be delayed. A number of factors may come into play in causing a girl's period to be "late"; extreme thinness, serious illness, poor nutritional practices, and even the mother's age at menarche may be involved. Some physically active girls who have trained heavily prior to and throughout adolescence may not get their first period until they are in their late teens or even early twenties. This absence of menarche may also be accompanied by a lack of secondary sex characteristics, such as the development of breasts and body hair.

Effects of Physical Activity

Researchers have been studying the link between heavy physical activity and delayed menarche for several years. One of the original theories on delayed menarche in physically active girls was developed by Dr. Rose Frisch at the Harvard Center for Population Studies. Dr. Frisch's hypothesis was that a girl had to reach a certain weight for her particular height before her periods would begin. In their study of young ballet dancers Dr. Frisch and her colleagues also took body composition into account. They knew that estrogen—a key hormone in the menstruation cycle—is activated and stored in fatty tissues. They therefore theorized that specific amounts of body fat were necessary for menarche to occur, and predicted that periods would begin when a girl reached a body composition of about 17 percent fat. This theory maintained that very thin or very physically active girls may not be reaching a high enough percent body fat for menstruation to begin.

While it is now generally accepted that a certain amount of body fat is necessary for menarche to occur, some researchers doubt that there is a particular body fat percentage or exact weight/height ratio at which menstrual cycles begin. Efforts have focused on various inconsistencies with the body fat theory. For example, a study of body composition and sexual maturation of adolescent athletes and nonathletes, conducted by Plowman et al. at the University of Arizona, concluded that "sexual maturation is not related to percent body fat in either premenarcheal athletes or non-athletes and is not impaired in athletes." Consider also that measurement of body fat, especially in children, is an inexact science. Other possibilities, such as diet or exercise patterns prior to menarche, are still being explored as contributors to menstrual patterns and menarche, and are equally acceptable in explaining the delay of menses.

So, why is it that athletes tend to have late menarche? In their 1994 letter to the editor of *Lancet*, Adam Baxter-Jones et al., researchers at the University of Aberdeen Scotland and the University of London, suggest from their longitudinal study of young British athletes that girls who mature later or are naturally thin or lean may be more prone to involvement in sports. For example, girls who are petite or tall or thin may pursue or be encouraged toward running, gymnastics, or ballet—sports that require a certain amount of leanness for success.

Dietary Needs

Puberty is a time of skeletal growth, due to an increase in the hormones estrogen and progestin. However, when menarche is late, those hormones may not be produced in quantities sufficient for pubertal development to fully occur. Prolonged delays in menarche may keep a girl from attaining her full skeletal mass later in life, resulting in thinning of the bones, and ultimately increasing her risk for osteoporosis. Unfortunately, these factors go unnoticed by many girls and their parents, because athletic adolescents or teens appear very fit, with muscular physiques and great cardiovascular fitness.

To understand how bones become "thin," it helps to know something about the way our bones grow. Bones are constantly undergoing a process of buildup and breakdown (resorption). Estrogen, the hormone that increases with menarche, is one of the factors that slow bone resorption so bones can have a chance to become thicker, stronger, and thus more resistant to fractures. The teens and twenties are prime times for a woman to build her skeleton to its peak. To help bolster this bone-building process, a girl with delayed periods may want to increase her dietary calcium. She should also take into account that some foods, such as caffeine present in soft drinks, chocolate, tea, and coffee, can actually increase calcium excretion in urine. One way to counteract this effect is to eat a balanced diet with plenty of calcium-rich foods.

When to Seek Help

Putting a timetable on when menarche should start could be a source of worry to many girls. A more sensible approach might be to look at all the various factors that could impact menarche. Is a girl training intensely in her sport? Is she eating well? Is she maintaining or gaining weight as she grows? What about levels of stress and general health? All these factors may play a part in delaying menarche.

Up to a certain point, we advise girls and their parents to let nature take its course, and accept a certain amount of lateness as natural for that girl. However, if a girl has not exhibited any secondary sex characteristics by about age 14, or has not experienced any menstrual cycles by age 16, she might want to consult with her health-care provider.

SHORTENED LUTEAL PHASE
AND LACK OF OVULATION

"When my running mileage was higher, my periods were much lighter and occurred less often. I suspect that I was not ovulating during those times, but never took my temperature to confirm it."

If you have ever been intensely active for a period of time (when training for a big event, for instance), you might have noticed a progression of changes from regular menstrual functioning to menstrual irregularity. At first, perhaps you had less intense premenstrual symptoms or a light flow. If you experienced the next steps in the progression—luteal phase defect and anovulation—chances are you may not have noticed them.

Luteal phase defect shortens the length of time between ovulation and the onset of bleeding, a phase that would normally take 14 days. In the case of anovulation, the cycle progresses normally, but no egg is released. The most serious consequences of these menstrual irregularities may be for the woman who is trying to conceive. Certainly if a woman does not ovulate month after month, she will not become pregnant. A woman experiencing shortened luteal phases may also experience fertility difficulties. There is also some concern about possible health risks associated with these conditions, because certain types of anovulation may involve some lowering of estrogen levels. Prolonged instances may result in some loss of bone mass. Keep in mind, however, that estrogen levels may be only slightly lowered by these conditions, and that other causes may also be contributing to lower bone density.

Effects of Physical Activity

Shortened luteal phase and lack of ovulation are considered initial steps on a continuum of menstrual cycle irregularity associated with physical activity. They may be only temporary conditions, or, depending on a variety of factors, they may progress toward menstrual cycle irregularity.

What causes these changes, and how do you know if you will be affected? This is a difficult question to answer, as every woman is different; however, your training patterns may be the best indicator. Menstrual cycle changes seem to be closely associated with sudden changes in physical activity patterns—specifically, sudden large increases in time, intensity, or distance. For example, if you have been taking one aerobics class a week for the past several years, and decide to take five classes a week and add some weight training another 2 days a week, your menstrual cycle might change as a result.

Your body may also be an indicator of your likeliness to develop shortened luteal phase or anovulation. If you are thin or have low body fat stores, you may be more prone to these conditions than a heavier woman with higher levels of body fat. In addition, the high energy expenditure associated with a dramatic increase in training may cause enough weight loss or loss of body fat to affect your menstrual cycle.

Detecting These Conditions

Some women don't realize they have luteal phase defect or anovulation because the overall length or nature of their cycle doesn't change dramatically. To actually measure the length of your luteal phase, you need to know if and when you ovulate. Taking your basal body temperature each morning for several months can help you pinpoint ovulation. If you do, it is important to take temperature readings before getting out of bed in the morning—before activity causes your body temperature to rise. Charting these temperatures on paper will allow you to see a visual trend over the month. Generally your temperature will be under 98 degrees F during the first part of your cycle, or follicular phase. Just before ovulation, your temperature will dip, and then it will rise over the next day or two. Throughout the second part, or luteal phase, your temperature will be above 98 degrees F. If your temperature does not fluctuate at all or fluctuates widely, you might not be ovulating.

In addition to charting, you might find it helpful to note physical changes such as pain and tenderness in the pelvic area that occur during the middle of your cycle. Cervical mucus will become thinner, more copious, and clear just before and during ovulation. Usually, if you have not ovulated, you will also not have premenstrual symptoms such as breast tenderness, mood changes, or bloating.

Laura took her basal body temperatures for 4 months to determine if she was ovulating. She was trying to become pregnant and had heard that as a long-distance runner, she might have problems conceiving. Laura found that the cyclic changes in her cervical mucus coincided with her temperature charts, indicating that she was ovulating each month. For the first 12 days of her cycle, the discharge was whitish and somewhat thick. As ovulation approached and before her temperature rose, it became thinner and clear for several days. Some months, Laura also had a light pain in her lower abdomen, indicating that she had ovulated. Laura needed to use the chart for only 4 months; since then, she's been able to tell if she's ovulating by paying attention to the physical signs.

On the following page is a chart you can use for keeping basal body temperatures. Day 1 of the chart should correspond to the first day of your menstrual flow. The numbers along the left side represent tenths of a degree in temperature. To record each day's temperature, place a dot at the point where the lines for the temperature and the day

Basal Body Temperature Chart

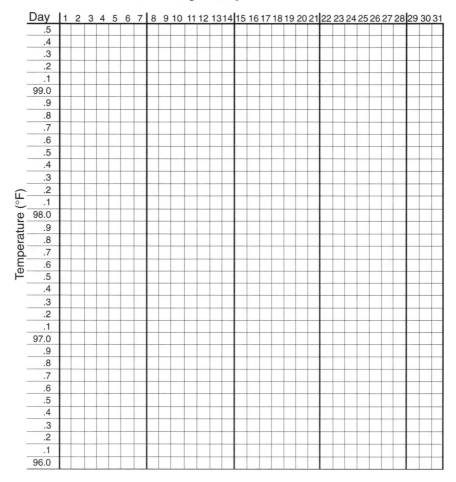

intersect. Calendar dates may be placed along the top of the chart for ease of recording.

A single month of charting is not enough to give you an accurate picture of your normal menstrual cycle. If you are trying to detect anovulation or shortened luteal phase, you'll want to keep records for several months. If you do find a pattern of irregularity, the next question is, "How long should I wait before I consult a doctor?"

When to Seek Help

While menstrual irregularity may be a natural response, it may not feel comfortable to you, especially if it interferes with your plans to get pregnant. If obvious menstrual changes and irregularities have been continuing for many months, we feel it is wise to consult your health-care provider. A few months of charted records will be useful in the consultations, especially if you are trying to become pregnant. Most physicians will begin fertility workups after a couple has been trying unsuccessfully to become pregnant for one year. Keeping temperature charts or a menstrual cycle diary may help determine the possible cause of infertility, saving time and money by avoiding the need for other diagnostic testing.

What can you expect in terms of treatment? Many researchers and physicians believe that menstrual irregularities are reversible through changes in training and lifestyle. A first step might be to decrease training time, intensity, or training patterns. A day or two off from training each week may be enough to regulate an irregular cycle. It may also be that your specific activity is affecting your cycle more than other activities would. If you are a runner, for instance, your doctor may ask you to substitute swimming or cycling for a while to see if that affects your menstrual pattern. He or she may also ask you to gain a moderate amount of weight through a sensible, nutritious diet. Before you begin any treatment plan, be sure to ask questions and become aware of all your options so you can make the best decision concerning your health.

ABSENCE OF MENSTRUAL PERIODS

"I feel healthy, but it worries me that I am not having a period."

"I just wanted to know why I wasn't getting my periods and if it was something to be concerned about."

"When I began running regularly I was on birth control pills and had regular periods. Since going off the pill I have only had a couple of light periods in 4-1/2 years."

"I was worried at first about not getting my period."

Perhaps the most disconcerting menstrual change for the physically active woman is that of athletic amenorrhea, or the absence of men-strual periods. The concept of "athletic amenorrhea," or the absence of menstrual periods associated with physical activity, moved into the spotlight during the fitness boom of the 1970s. As more women became physically active, interest and research in this area accelerated. Reports of the possible connection between loss of periods and exercise alarmed many women who were already exercising and deterred others from starting a physical activity program.

Since then, pinpointing the exact cause of athletic amenorrhea has been the focus for many researchers and the topic of numerous studies. It is apparent that there is no single cause of athletic amenorrhea, but actually a combination of many factors. At first, researchers suspected that thinness combined with intense activity may be primarily responsible. Today, researchers are also looking at the role of the hypothalamus, an organ at the base of the brain that controls the glandular systems in the body. Hypothalamic rhythm may be altered by intense physical training, perhaps as a way for the body to conserve energy. It may be that these glandular changes cause the body to produce fewer ovary-stimulating hormones; in turn, the ovary produces less estrogen. Lower estrogen could be one of the many factors that cause amenorrhea or oligomenorrhea (infrequent periods). Body fat, nutrition, and even stress can also exert an influence on menstrual cycles, making it difficult for us to say for sure which is responsible for irregularities.

Body Fat and Body Weight

"I quit menstruating right after a combination of weight loss and also starting endurance activity on a regular basis."

"It seems my cycle stops under stress—a weight gain or loss of more than 5 pounds, pressure from work, or travel."

As a result of early research, physicians and athletes are sometimes quick to blame low body weight and low body fat for the loss of periods. However, in 1985, Charlotte Sanborn, Bruce Albrecht, and Wiltz Wagner, Jr., at the University of Colorado upset this notion. They compared women who had athletic amenorrhea with women who were menstruating regularly. The two groups were similar in age, height, weight, and training levels. It is of interest that the women in both of these groups also had similar body fat percentages.

Some researchers speculate that the distribution of body fat may have a greater influence on reproductive function than simply how much body fat we have. Researcher Kelly Brownell, at Yale University, suggests that certain fat deposits are necessary to provide energy for both pregnancy and lactation. In humans, this lactational fat is found on the hips, thighs, and buttocks. When these fat stores are depleted, as in high levels of physical training, menstrual dysfunction may result.

Nutrition

"I continued running, but added a little fat to my diet. My periods resumed within 6 months."

"My family eats a very low-fat, mostly vegetarian diet, and maybe I am not ingesting enough protein or fat, which might be contributing to my menstrual irregularity."

At Melpomene, we were interested in finding out what part nutrition plays in the maintenance of menstrual periods. We asked groups of amenorrheic and regularly menstruating athletes to keep track of their diets as well as their physical activity patterns. We found that the amenorrheic athletes ate an average of 450 calories less per day than regularly menstruating athletes. The interesting thing was that these women seemed to be able to maintain their weight on this lowered intake.

We suspect that this may be due to the phenomenon of food efficiency. Food efficiency is an adaptive process whereby the body adjusts to lower caloric intakes by making the most of the calories it is given. People with enhanced food efficiency can function and maintain their current weight even though they seem to be eating too little. For example, Andrea weighs 120 pounds, rows 2 hours each day, and consumes 2,500 calories daily. Barbara also weighs 120 pounds and consumes 2,500 calories daily, but rows 4 hours each day. Both Andrea and Barbara are maintaining their current weight of 120 pounds. Barbara is more food efficient, however, because she is able to maintain her weight, eating the same as Andrea, despite her much higher level of caloric expenditure through rowing.

Brownell speculates that food efficiency may be an adaptive trait in human beings, designed to carry a person through a biologically taxing time (e.g., famine). He and his colleagues state:

For theoretical reasons, we would expect food efficiency to be enhanced in athletes with low or fluctuating weights. These patterns may be perceived as a threat to energy stores, thus increased efficiency could be the defense. The effect should be most pronounced in athletes who are furthest below their non-training weight. The effect may be stronger in females than males because their reproductive function is more readily threatened by changes in energy stores.

When a cave woman had to survive a winter of low food rations, for example, it would be beneficial for her metabolism to slow down so

Nutritional Tips to Resume Menstruation and Reduce the Risks of Amenorrhea

Nancy Clark, MS, RD, of Nutrition Services at SportsMedicine Brookline in Boston, provides the following nutritional tips to resume menses or reduce the risks of amenorrhea:

1. Cut back your exercise by 5 to 15 percent.
2. Increase your caloric consumption.
3. Eat on a regular schedule. Include wholesome, balanced meals that provide adequate nutrients and energy.
4. Make sure you are eating an adequate amount of protein. (Clark notes that .5 gram to .75 gram of protein per pound of body weight is recommended for exercising women and is a higher amount than that recommended for sedentary women.)
5. Vegetarian diets may lack protein. Including red meat in meals two to three times per week is important for athletic women. Runners with amenorrhea tend to show the absence of red meat in their diets, and many follow vegetarian diets. Due to recent concern over fat in red meat, Americans fear eating fat, but it is still possible to include lean red meat in the diet in smaller portions. This is especially true for athletes' low-fat diets.
6. Twenty percent of calories from fat is a minimum requirement for athletes. Eating 40 to 60 grams of fat per day provides a balance in an athlete's or regular exerciser's diet. Beef, peanut butter, and nuts are examples of nutrient-rich foods that are higher in fat.
7. Eating a calcium-rich diet provides some protection against bone loss and osteoporosis. Guidelines include 800 to 1,200 milligrams of calcium per day as a minimum for exercising women.

Adapted, by permission, from N. Clark, 1993, "Athletes with Amenorrhea," *The Physician and Sportsmedicine* 21 (4), 45-46.

that she could survive on less food. Perhaps the body interprets intense exercise as another kind of environmental stress. It makes good biological sense not to bring a child into the world when food shortages are low and energy outputs are high; pregnancy and lactation simply take too much energy. In this light, the disruption of periods can also be seen as an adaptive/protective response to stress.

On the average, the women in our study who were the most food efficient were also amenorrheic. Other studies on athletes and nutrition have concurred with our findings, pointing to the need for pregnant women to consume an adequate number of calories if they want to maintain general good health while meeting the increased energy needs of physical training.

Vegetarianism has also been studied for its possible link to athletic amenorrhea. Many researchers, including Susan M. Brooks et al., at the University of Colorado; Patricia A. Deuster et al., at the University of Maryland; and Karl M. Pirke et al., in a West German study, have found a high number of vegetarians among the amenorrheic athletes whom they study. In our study, 85 percent of the amenorrheic women said they did not eat red meat; only 25 percent of the regularly menstruating women made the same statement. Some researchers feel that vegetarianism may affect the hormones that influence the menstrual cycle in two ways. First, these women may not be getting enough dietary fat, which is important for estrogen production and storage. Second, it is possible that vegetarian women eat more fiber than non-vegetarian women, and so are more likely to excrete estrogen in their feces. Another relevant finding from the Melpomene study was that the amenorrheic women were eating three to four times more vitamin A than the regularly menstruating women were eating. Beta carotene, which is a form of vitamin A found in plants and vegetables, is stored in fat cells and in the corpus luteum (in the ovaries). Researchers hypothesize that the excessive levels of beta carotene in the fat cells of very lean women may interfere with estrogen production. It is also possible that high levels of deposited beta carotene in the ovaries of these women may affect their menstrual cycles.

Physical Activity

"When I injured my knee and had to stop running for a while, menstruation returned."

"I have cut back a little on the number of miles I run each week."

It may not be how long or how intensely you work out that causes a change in your menstrual cycle. The real disruption seems to occur when you change your level of activity abruptly. A woman who goes from doing nothing to running several miles a day, for instance, may be more likely to develop menstrual problems than the woman who slowly works up to that level of activity.

The sport in which you choose to participate may also affect your menstrual patterns. Studies have shown that there is a higher incidence of amenorrhea in "thin person" sports than in sports in which weight does not matter. Menstrual problems are found to be common, for instance, in women who participate in distance running, ballet, and gymnastics. In contrast, swimmers have a fairly low incidence of amenorrhea or menstrual changes. This is partly due to the higher levels of body fat that swimmers maintain for regulating body temperature in the water.

Very high levels of training have also been found to be a factor in athletic amenorrhea, especially during dramatic increases in training levels. Over time, the body may adapt to the higher levels of activity, but initially the high energy expenditure and possible lowering of body weight/fat may be enough to disrupt periods.

The Effects of Long-Term Athletic Amenorrhea

"What concerns me is prolonged amenorrhea. I am married and may someday be interested in having children and am curious if this will present problems."

Two questions most women ask about their own amenorrhea are "Is it harmful to me?" and "Will it affect my fertility?" For many years, scientists and physicians were divided as to the long-term effects of athletic amenorrhea. Then in the early 1980s researchers found that athletes who did not have menstrual periods seemed to be losing mineral content in their bones, which may put them at risk for osteoporosis. The phenomenon of bone tissue loss is normal and occurs in each of us, but it is usually offset by bone buildup—a balance that keeps our bones strong. One of the key ingredients in this balance is estrogen, the hormone that controls the rate of bone loss through resorption. Without estrogen to slow bone loss, the balance was thrown out of whack, and the athletes studied began seeing a net loss in bone density, especially in the spine. This was somewhat surprising considering that muscle activity through exercise is known to actually increase total bone mass. Evidently, exercise was not enough to offset the bone loss caused by lowered estrogen. The longer a woman experiences amenorrhea, the longer her body has decreased levels of estrogen, resulting in a loss of bone density and an increased risk of osteoporosis in later life.

Bone loss due to athletic amenorrhea can be a problem for athletes of all ages. Girls with primary amenorrhea (who have never menstruated) may not undergo normal pubertal bone growth in the same way as other girls who have normal, regular periods. Therefore, they may not experience normal skeletal growth, and the result is a failure to obtain peak skeletal maturity. Adolescents with secondary amenorrhea (who have reached menarche, but have stopped menstruating since then) run the same risk as those who have never had a period. However, girls with secondary amenorrhea tend to respond better to treatments involving a decrease in exercise or training habits and dietary changes, reversing amenorrhea more rapidly than adolescents who have never had a period. The sooner cycles start or are resumed, the greater opportunity for bone density and bone mineral content to increase.

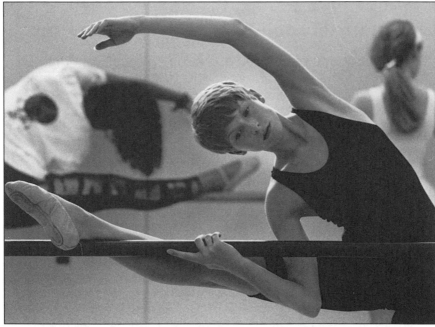

Courtesy of the *Daily Illini*

Girls with primary amenorrhea may not experience normal skeletal growth—the result is a failure to obtain peak skeletal maturity.

Bone loss is also apparent in menopausal women, who may lose up to 2 percent of their bone mass per year for the first 4 to 5 years after menopause. The rate of bone loss continues in the later postmenopausal years, but usually at a slower rate. The loss of estrogen is also the cause of bone loss in premenopausal women who have had their ovaries removed.

On the positive side, Dr. Barbara Drinkwater of the Pacific Medical Center in Seattle, one of the early researchers to explore the link between bone loss and amenorrhea, conducted a study of amenorrheic women who had resumed their menstrual cycles. She found that their bone density increased after their cycles began again. However, her more recent research concludes that while some of bone density lost may be made up, this gain may be limited. Drinkwater finds that women with menstrual irregularities are ultimately left with less bone density than those women who have always had regular menstrual cycles. Therefore, it is important that athletic amenorrhea, especially prolonged episodes, be discussed with your health-care provider. This may be especially true for the older amenorrheic athlete, since she is not as readily able to rebuild lost bone density after about age 35.

A second concern for the amenorrheic athlete is fertility. Many women who have stopped having periods are worried that they won't be able to get pregnant. While it's true that you can't get pregnant if you are not ovulating, it's also true that amenorrhea can reverse itself at any time. You may skip your period for 3 months and then suddenly ovulate and menstruate in the fourth month.

Once a woman starts ovulating and menstruating again, the fact that she was once amenorrheic does not seem to have any effect on her fertility. As long as she starts ovulating at mid-cycle, she is capable of conceiving children. Amenorrhea, like an oral contraceptive, merely causes a time out in reproductive functioning. Once that is reversed, regular reproductive functioning should resume. (Because you can't predict when ovulation might resume again, it's not a good idea to use amenorrhea as a form of birth control!)

If you are having regular periods after having been amenorrheic, and you are still unable to get pregnant, it may be that you are not ovulating mid-cycle. Outwardly, your cycle can seem completely normal, but if you don't release an egg, you won't be able to get pregnant. It is also common to experience infrequent periods in the transition from amenorrhea to regular cycles. Charting basal body temperatures will help you to determine if you are ovulating. Again, this is a helpful tool when consulting your physician about fertility problems.

Treatment

"I had one period last year, and it was brought on by the use of prescribed drugs."

"I am willing to slow down the running; so far I've been replacing it with more swimming."

"I have not had a period in 4 years and have cut back on my jogging. My doctor thinks estrogen/progesterone will help. I don't really care to take these hormones. Help!"

"My concern now is to regain a normal menstrual cycle so I can become pregnant. I have stopped running entirely for almost a year now. I have also increased my weight from a low of 100 pounds 3 years ago to 112 pounds at present."

"I would like to become pregnant. I would also like not to have to give up those 40 or 50 miles per week running."

"I am currently being seen by an ob/gyn who put me on birth control pills about 6 months ago. They seem to be working well. I'm having regular periods after 6-1/2 years of nothing!"

Many women who develop athletic amenorrhea are not sure what to do. Some feel it is imperative to see their physician as soon as they miss a period, and others are willing to wait several months or even a year before consulting a doctor. This timetable is a matter of personal choice. However, to rule out other causes of amenorrhea, including pregnancy or pituitary malfunctions, we feel it is important to check with your physician after one missed period if you suspect pregnancy. Otherwise, most physicians feel that you should consult your doctor after three missed periods.

When it comes to treating athletic amenorrhea, the experts fall into two camps. Some feel that it is important to treat amenorrhea immediately to avoid possible problems with bone demineralization or fertility. Others have a wait-and-see attitude. They believe that athletic amenorrhea is the body's way of adapting to the extra stresses of physical training, lower caloric consumption, or a change in body composition. They contend that in most cases, amenorrhea will reverse itself without intervention. When consulting your physician about amenorrhea, make sure he or she performs the following procedures to determine the cause before beginning any sort of treatment plan.

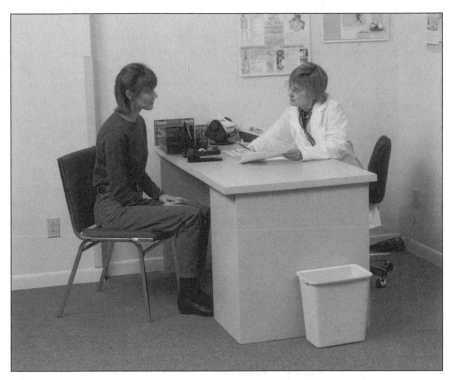

If you suspect pregnancy might be the cause of amenorrhea, consult your physician after one missed period.

1. Collect or update your health information and history. This should include a history of dieting or weight loss, amount and intensity of exercise, a nutritional assessment, and any past health and reproductive problems. Psychological factors such as stress should also be considered, as well as the possibility of anorexia nervosa or other eating disorders.
2. Perform a pelvic exam to observe any reproductive abnormalities or possible pregnancy.
3. If everything appears normal and you are not pregnant, he or she should order some laboratory studies that will determine your levels of hormones such as plasma prolactin. Prolactin, which is important for lactation, has been found to increase in some highly trained athletic women, and researchers believe the increase may be associated with athletic amenorrhea. Your doctor should also know about any medications you are taking, since certain medications can elevate prolactin levels. Thyroid levels should also be measured to rule out hypothyroidism

(underactive thyroid). If prolactin is elevated, then a CT scan may be necessary to see if a pituitary tumor exists.

4. At the same time, your physician will probably perform what is called a Provera challenge to determine if your levels of estrogen are low. This involves your taking Provera for 7 to 10 days and waiting for about 3 days to see if you have withdrawal bleeding. If you do bleed, this means that you have sufficient levels of estrogen to build up the lining of your uterus. However, if you do not bleed, your estrogen levels are probably decreased, and your physician may want to perform further laboratory tests, such as measuring levels of FSH and LH.

5. Finally, if you've been amenorrheic for a long time, he or she might want to make an estimate of your bone density before developing a treatment plan.

After all these tests, you and your physician may choose to do nothing while waiting to see if your periods resume naturally. Your doctor might also recommend that you trim back your training schedule, do a different activity once or twice a week (such as tennis or swimming instead of running), or eliminate speed training for a few months. Your physician may also suggest that you gain some weight. A regimen of decreased training and weight gain is not guaranteed to produce immediate results, however; it may still take several months before your period returns, or you may discover that this change in activity level or weight gain does not improve your ability to conceive. Many athletes may find it difficult and unappealing to reduce their training program or increase their body weight. However, reducing the amount of exercise and increasing body weight are two approaches that may make a difference in your menstrual cycle patterns.

Another treatment for athletic amenorrhea is hormonal replacement therapy. Estrogen and/or progesterone, possibly in the form of birth control pills, may be prescribed to treat amenorrhea and to prevent bone loss. If side effects or health risks do not make this option sensible, the following regimes may be suggested by your health-care professional. In most cases, you will take 5 to 10 milligrams per day of medroxyprogesterone (Amen, Provera) for 10 days each cycle and/or .625 milligram per day of conjugated estrogens (Premarin) for days 1 through 25 of a cycle to prevent bone demineralization. If you have withdrawal bleeding after taking these hormones, you'll know that your outflow tract (uterus and vagina) is normal.

Again, you and your health-care provider must make a choice from among treatment options. Be sure your physician is willing to answer your questions, listen to your concerns, and present and discuss all the options before you begin treatment. The success of a treatment depends on your makeup and health history; what works wonders for a friend of yours may not be appropriate for you. It's especially important to think carefully about hormonal replacement treatments. If you do choose to work with hormones, both you and your physician should pay close attention to any changes or side effects that may occur.

PREMENSTRUAL SYNDROME (PMS)

"Usually, the day before I get my period I have extreme highs and lows in my mood."

"I get irritable and emotional 2-3 days before I begin menstruating."

"Two weeks before the onset of my period, I have severe melancholy and lethargy. Getting my period is a relief."

"I am inclined to binge on chocolate prior to my flow if I'm not paying attention."

"I'm much more active in the summer and I notice significantly fewer mood swings and less physical pain around menstruation."

Many women go through cyclical changes a few days before their period. Their moods may fluctuate, their breasts may be sore, or perhaps they feel bloated with a few extra pounds of "water weight." For 10 percent of all menstruating women, these physical and psychological changes can be severe enough to disrupt their lives. Premenstrual syndrome, or PMS, is experienced by 40 percent of all women who menstruate. Despite its prevalence, PMS is still the subject of much controversy in the medical community. Scientists and physicians can't seem to agree on an exact definition, or even whether PMS is a discrete syndrome. One problem is that the symptoms are so wide-ranging that it's difficult to tie them to a single syndrome. And although some treatments work for some symptoms (e.g., nutritional therapies can ease depression), there is no treatment for PMS that is consistently effective for all symptoms.

No one really knows what causes PMS. Some researchers believe that hormonal change or imbalance is the culprit. One popular theory is that PMS is linked to an imbalance in the ratio of progesterone to estrogen. It is also possible that PMS is actually more than one syndrome, with different causes for each symptom or group of symptoms. This theory would explain why no single treatment is effective for all symptoms or all women.

In general, PMS occurs every month and is cyclical in nature. Symptoms appear during the luteal phase (last half) of the cycle and should lessen once the menstrual period begins. Then at least one symptom-free week should occur. Note that PMS should not be confused with dysmenorrhea, which is characterized by pain and cramping during menstrual periods.

Symptoms

PMS encompasses a wide range of symptoms, both physical and psychological. Bloating is the most common physical symptom, but breast tenderness, swelling, pelvic pain, headache, and bowel changes are also prevalent. Irritability and aggressiveness are some of the most common psychological symptoms of PMS. Others include depression, anxiety, lack of concentration, appetite changes, tension, change in sex drive, and insomnia.

A good way to determine if you suffer from PMS is to chart your symptoms. Keeping a menstrual calendar or chart like the one on page 170 can help you determine which symptoms are cyclic, when they occur, and whether they are in fact premenstrual. A chart should include (1) the days you menstruate, (2) the days that symptoms occur, (3) the symptom, and (4) the severity of the symptom. Recording your basal body temperature each day (see page 154) can be especially helpful in determining when you ovulate and when you are premenstrual. You might also find it useful to keep track of your physical activity levels and how you feel on certain days of your cycle in relation to your exercise program.

After 3 or 4 months of charting, you may see patterns emerge that will help you identify your problem and target your treatment. Try grouping the symptoms that you see cropping up into either physical or psychological categories (e.g., bloating and breast tenderness would be physical symptoms, while anxiety, depression, and frequent crying would be psychological). If symptoms are disabling or severe enough to be interfering with your life, and you do seek medical help, this grouping will help your physician prescribe the most effective treatment for you.

Watching Your PMT

Below is a scheme for categorizing PMS symptoms as proposed by endocrinologist Dr. Guy Abraham. The initials PMT (Premenstrual Tension) are followed by A for anxiety, C for carbohydrate craving and intolerance, H for hyper-hydration or water retention, and D for depression.

PMTA (Anxiety) Affects 80 Percent of PMS Sufferers
  Nervous tension
  Mood swings
  Irritability
  Anger
  Anxiety
  Depression
PMTC (Carbohydrate Craving and Intolerance)
Affects 60 Percent of PMS Sufferers
  Headache
  Sweet cravings
  Alcohol cravings
  Increased appetite
  Heart pounding
  Fatigue
  Dizziness
  Faintness
PMTH (Hyper-Hydration or Water Retention)
Affects 40 Percent of PMS Sufferers
  Weight gain
  Swelling of extremities
  Breast tenderness
  Abdominal bloating
PMTD (Depression) Affects 20 Percent of PMS Suffers
  Severe depression
  Withdrawal
  Confusion
  Crying easily
  Insomnia
  Forgetfulness
  Suicidal thoughts

Premenstrual Symptoms Chart

Grading of Symptoms

0 None
1 Mild: present but does not interfere with activities
2 Moderate: present and interferes with activities but
   not disabling
3 Severe: disabling, unable to function

Date	1	2	3	4	5	6	7	8	9	10	11	12	13	14	15	16	17	18	19	20	21	22	23	24	25	26	27	28	29	30	31
Basal weight																															
Basal body temp																															
Menstruation																															
Day of cycle																															
Nervous tension																															
Mood swings																															
Irritability																															
Anxiety																															
Headache																															
Cravings																															
Increased appetite																															
Nausea																															
Depression																															
Forgetfulness																															
Crying																															
Confusion																															
Clumsiness																															
Insomnia																															
Weight gain																															
Swelling																															
Breast tenderness																															
Bloating																															
Cramps																															
Backache																															
Aches & pains																															
Diarrhea																															
Constipation																															
Skin changes																															
Allergies																															
Infections																															
Other symptoms:																															
Treatments:																															
Physical activity:																															

Adapted, by permission, from the Women's Health Clinic, Winnepeg, Manitoba, Canada.

Treatment

While many of the women affected by PMS do not need treatment, some are debilitated by symptoms each month. For these women, treatment may significantly improve the quality of their lives. Drug therapies for PMS include hormonal interventions, antianxiety agents, antidepressants, and diuretics. However, because of the possibility of adverse side effects associated with any prescription medication, women should consider any of these therapies only after other treatments have not worked. Nonprescription treatments range from diet or vitamin therapy to stress reduction exercises and massage.

Most experts agree that physical activity can have some value in relieving PMS symptoms. Dr. Jerilyn Prior at the University of British Columbia found that stress and anxiety were decreased in groups of women who had begun exercise, or who had increased training levels. The women in the study who were not training did not experience these improvements.

Researchers are also pointing to the kind of exercise that is more likely to relieve premenstrual symptoms. John Steege and James Blumenthal at Duke University Medical Center in Durham, North Carolina, found that women who engaged in aerobic exercise experienced a decrease in more premenstrual symptoms, especially premenstrual depression, than women who engaged in a strength-training program.

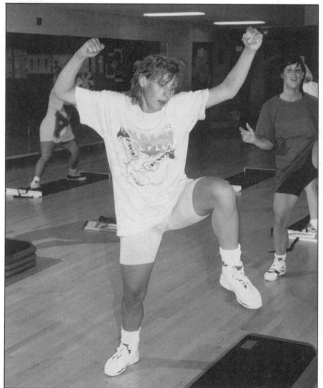

© David R. Barnes

Researchers offer several possible explanations for why aerobic exercise seems to alleviate premenstrual symptoms.

Aerobic activity, in which the heart rate is increased, may alleviate PMS symptoms better than non-aerobic activity because the increase in circulation associated with aerobic exercise can decrease bloating and fluid buildup. Also, the beta-endorphins responsible for "runner's high" can help lighten or calm your mood. Australian researchers Julie Aganoff and Gregory Boyle support this hypothesis. They found that women who exercise regularly showed decreased levels of "negative mood states," such as anger or sadness. They suggest that improvements in body image and self-esteem may have an impact on negative moods associated with PMS. They also speculate that the positive thoughts and distraction that regular exercise offers may alleviate symptoms. Physical activity may also enhance relaxation by relieving muscular tension and helping to lessen joint pain. Finally, regular exercise increases the effectiveness of insulin, which helps your body convert starches and sugars into energy. This fast and efficient digestion helps stabilize blood sugar levels and decrease food cravings during the premenstrual stage.

CONTRACEPTION

"I am concerned about putting on weight if I go on the pill. I am also worried about the emotional side effects."

"I have found that barrier methods of contraception have had the least impact on my physical activities."

"I have been using oral contraceptives for over 10 years and have not experienced any menstrual irregularities as a result of running. Will either one make it any easier or more difficult for me to conceive, if and when I choose to do so?"

Most physically active women are health-conscious and committed to making decisions that enhance their health and well-being. Women faced with contraceptive choices are often undecided as to which method is best for them. Most women are looking for a safe, effective method of contraception that poses no health risks and will not jeopardize future fertility. Women who are active may be concerned with how side effects will affect their athletic endeavors, or how birth control devices will stand up to the rigors of intense activity.

In a 1990 survey of 672 Melpomene members, we asked about contraceptive choice. We were interested in learning more about what contraceptive practices physically active women choose and whether those choices have any relationship to or effect on physical activity.

For respondents of this survey, barrier methods, in the form of condoms and the diaphragm, were the first two ranking choices of contraception. However, when we divided the respondents into groups by level of physical activity—women who were physically active for 4 hours or more a week (active) and those who were physically active for less than 4 hours a week (less active)—we found some noticeable differences. For the less active group, the first two ranking choices of contraception were still condoms and the diaphragm; however, for the active group, condom use was followed by partner vasectomy as the top two choices. Also, diaphragm use was less among active respondents (active, 17.1 percent; less active, 22.3 percent), and oral contraceptives (birth control pills) were used more often among the active group (active, 13.9 percent; less active, 7.7 percent).

We also asked respondents to tell us about the effects, if any, their birth control method had on their physical activity. Most women reported being unaffected by their contraceptive choice. However, negative effects were most prevalent for the birth control pill, the diaphragm, and the IUD. Sterilization procedures produced the most positive effects. Partner vasectomy ranked first, followed by tubal ligation and abstinence.

Barrier Methods

More and more physically active women are choosing barrier methods of contraception, such as condoms, the diaphragm, cervical cap, or contraceptive foam or jelly. Barrier methods give the woman more control over contraception with minimal side effects. Also, barrier methods do not interfere with the body's hormonal system, nor with physical activity for the most part. Diaphragms, however, must be left in for 6 hours after intercourse and may therefore need to be left in during exercise. Some Melpomene members commented that exercising with a diaphragm in place can be painful and cause uterine cramping or even urinary tract infections. One member wrote, "Sometimes I would run with the diaphragm in and it seemed to lead to urinary tract infections. It was also sometimes painful." Other members complained that diaphragm use was messy. One woman commented, "The only problem with the diaphragm is excessive discharge, which can be a problem during activities like running and cycling." While the "messiness" associated with diaphragm use during exercise may not be avoided, a smaller-size diaphragm may alleviate the discomfort of exercising with the diaphragm in place.

Athletes tend to avoid using the intrauterine device (IUD) as a method of contraception. The IUD was the method of choice for only

2.9 percent of Melpomene members. Possible side effects associated with the IUD may deter physically active women from choosing this method. Complications associated with IUD use are heavier periods, dysmenorrhea, and an increased risk of pelvic inflammatory disease, particularly during the first few weeks after insertion, which may cause infertility. One woman described her experience: "I used the IUD for 2 years. Severe cramping and heavy bleeding basically curtailed physical activity for 5 to 7 days. It was awful!"

While the IUD may not be a choice for many women, it is a very effective means of contraception. In addition, one type—the Copper T380A—can be left in place for up to 10 years, making it a very inexpensive birth control method.

A newer option among barrier methods is the female condom. It provides protection by lining the vagina entirely and partially shielding the perineum. The female condom is inserted into the vagina with an inner ring that covers the cervix. It allows women to protect themselves against unwanted pregnancies and sexually transmitted diseases, including AIDS. Most other birth control options for women don't protect against these diseases. Some people seem to think the female condom is a strange option when considering birth control. However, with more exposure and educational efforts, more people may find it a comfortable contraceptive option. Also, while the female condom has not been tested by years of use, it should, like the male condom, pose few complications for the physically active woman.

Rhythm Method

The rhythm method of contraception requires the charting of basal body temperature and changes in cervical mucus in order to determine fertile times. Athletes who experience menstrual irregularities such as anovulatory cycles and shortened luteal phase will find that the rhythm method is unreliable. In the same way, amenorrhea is not an effective form of birth control. As we mentioned before, you never know when ovulation will occur.

Sterilization Methods

Sterilization methods have become an increasingly popular option for men and women who have chosen not to have children or who have completed their families. The members who chose sterilization reported few or no negative effects and a high number of positive effects. Vasectomies and tubal ligations are extremely effective and eliminate the worry and inconvenience associated with temporary forms of birth control. As one member stated, "The tubal was my choice. I did not want to be on hormones, and other things are too much fuss and bother. Now that it's done, I don't have to worry or do anything."

Oral Contraceptives

For many women, oral contraceptives or birth control pills provide a convenient option. There are two types of oral contraceptives: combination pills which contain both estrogen and progestin, and progestin-only pills. Birth control pills may present a real dilemma for women, because both benefits and risks are associated with their use. They are convenient, produce regular menstrual cycles, and often decrease dysmenorrhea. Oral contraceptives provide powerful protection against four gynecologic problems: ovarian cancer, endometrial cancer, ectopic pregnancy, and pelvic inflammatory disease. They also offer protection against iron-deficiency anemia, primary dysmenorrhea, benign breast disease, and functional ovarian cysts. Moreover, combination birth control pills provide enough estrogen to prevent bone loss in those women who are at risk.

Despite these advantages, the pill does have its share of negative side effects. In general, there is a four times greater risk of cardiovascular problems, deep vein thrombosis (blood clots), or stroke in women who take birth control pills than in non-pill users. Five out of every 100,000 women who use the pill die from these complications each year. The chance for problems increases with women who smoke, who are over age 35, and who have been on the pill for many years. For women under 35 years who do not smoke, the mortality rate falls to 0.7 per 100,000 women per year. For athletic women, the risks may be even lower due to lower body weight, lower body fat, and the fact that athletic women are aerobically conditioned—all factors that lower the risk of cardiovascular disease. Also, most physically active women do not smoke.

Concern regarding a potential association between oral contraceptives and malignant breast tumors dates as far back as when steroids first became available in the early 1960s. Over time, studies have focused on specific risk factors, such as age at first use of oral contraceptives, long-term use, use before first-term pregnancy, and use by both older and younger women. Although some widely reported recent studies have supported the hypothesis of increased risk of breast cancer with oral contraceptive use in specific subgroups, a larger number of studies have shown no significant increased risk. The jury is still out on the relationship between oral contraceptives and breast cancer. To date, nearly all studies have found that the incidence of breast cancer diagnosed in women 20 to 54 years old is the same for women who have ever used oral contraceptives as for women who have never used them. However, controversies still remain, such as whether the risk varies by age at breast cancer diagnosis.

Active women often want to know if birth control pills will affect their athletic performance. The research that has been conducted in this area is not conclusive. Some studies measuring maximum oxygen consumption ($\dot{V}O_2$ max), one measure of aerobic capacity, have reported a decrease in performance among oral contraceptive users. However, other research documenting the effects of oral contraceptives, using measures of fitness other than $\dot{V}O_2$ max, has found no differences between oral contraceptive users and nonusers. The possibility of side effects, such as weight gain due to water retention, is another reason some athletes steer away from the pill. However, newer, lower-dose oral contraceptives are continuing to gain in popularity, in part because they produce less fluid retention and weight gain than the earlier birth control pills did.

Other Hormonal Contraceptives

Women who are considering birth control pills now also have two other options; Depo-Provera and Norplant. Depo-Provera is an injectable progestin given to women every 3 months. It is a very effective method of birth control. Out of 1,000 women who use Depo-Provera, only three will become pregnant during the first year. The advantages of using Depo-Provera include convenience, in that it does not need to be taken daily or put in place before intercourse, and also its privacy. The injection ranges in cost from $22 to $40. The most common side effect of Depo-Provera is irregular bleeding. This may include longer menstrual flow, irregular intervals between periods, spotting between periods, or no bleeding for months at a time. Additionally it can take an average of 9 to 10 months for a woman to get pregnant after her last injection; for some, it may take up to 18 months to return to normal. Other side effects include change in appetite, weight gain, sore breasts, depression, and changes in sex drive.

Norplant is a reversible prescription method of birth control. Six soft capsules, each about the size of a cardboard matchstick, are inserted under the skin of the upper arm. Like any other progestin-only contraceptive (Depo-Provera and mini-pills), Norplant tends to cause menstrual irregularities. Bleeding usually becomes more regular after

9 to 12 months of use. A small number of women experience irregular bleeding throughout the 5 years which is the maximum amount of time that Norplant can remain in place. Other side effects with Norplant include headaches, changes in appetite, weight loss or gain, sore breasts, acne, enlarged ovaries, discolored skin over the implants, and pain experienced during insertion or removal. Norplant costs between $500 and $750 for the medical exam, the implants, and the insertion. An additional charge may be added for removal which can occur at any time during the 5 years. Advantages of Norplant include its convenience in providing long-lasting birth control and the fact that it does not need to be taken daily or put in place before intercourse.

Choosing the Best Method for You

The chart here summarizes the various contraceptive methods, as well as some of their advantages, disadvantages, and considerations for physical activity.

Considerations for Choosing a Contraceptive Method

Method	Pregnancy rate*	Implications for physical activity
Abstinence	0-0%	None
Coitus interruptus (withdrawal)	19.0-4.0	None
Postovulation method	20.0-1.0	None
Sympto-thermal method	20.0-2.0	None
Cervical mucus (ovulation) method	20.0-3.0	None
Calendar method	20.0-9.0	None
Sterilization		
Men	0.15-0.1	Physical activity restricted postoperatively (1 week-1 month)
Women	0.4-0.4	
Norplant	0.09-0.09	Irregular bleeding, weight changes possible

(cont.)

Considerations for Choosing a Contraceptive Method (cont.)

Method	Pregnancy rate*	Implications for physical activity
Depo-Provera	0.3-0.3	Irregular bleeding, weight changes possible
Combination birth control pills	3.0-0.1	Possible water weight increase, breast tenderness, pills may affect performance
Progestin-only birth control pills	3.0-0.5	Spotting between periods, pills may affect performance
Intrauterine device (IUD)		May cause pain and increased bleeding
Progesterone T	2.0-1.5	
Copper T380A	0.8-0.6	
Condom		
Men	12.0-3.0	None
Women	21.0-5.0	
Diaphragm	18.0-6.0	Discomfort possible, messy
Sponge		
Women who have not had a child	18.0-9.0	Currently off the market due to FDA updating
Women who have had a child	36.0-20.0	
Cervical cap		
Women who have not had a child	18.0-9.0	Discomfort possible, messy
Women who have had a child	36.0-26.0	
Foam, gel, film, and suppositories	21.0-6.0	Discharge, messy
No method	85.0-85.0	None

*Failure rate per 100 women per year. High number represents failure rate for one year of typical use. Low number represents theoretical failure rate for one year of perfect use, when a method is used correctly and consistently.

Data from Hatcher, R.A., and Trussell, J., et al. 1994. *Contraceptive Technology*, 16th ed. New York: Irvington.

In choosing a method of contraception, you will want to consider its effectiveness. Clearly, some forms of contraception are more effective than others. For example, some barrier methods can have a failure rate as high as 20 to 25 percent per 100 women per year of use, compared with a failure rate of 3 percent for birth control pills.

Whatever contraceptive method you decide on, we recommend that you consider not only its effectiveness, but also its impact on your health, lifestyle, and future fertility. In the final analysis, you are the best judge of what feels right to you, and therefore only you can make decisions about your health.

YOUR PERSONAL CYCLE

In this chapter, we've looked at the many changes, both major and minor, that can alter your menstrual cycle. On the one hand, physical activity can improve your health, but on the other hand, it may at some point affect your menstrual patterns. Other lifestyle factors such as diet and stress may also have an effect on your cycle. Keep in mind that while your cycle variations may not be average or what is considered "normal," these variations are not necessarily unhealthy, and may in fact be quite common among other women who are enjoying a physically active lifestyle.

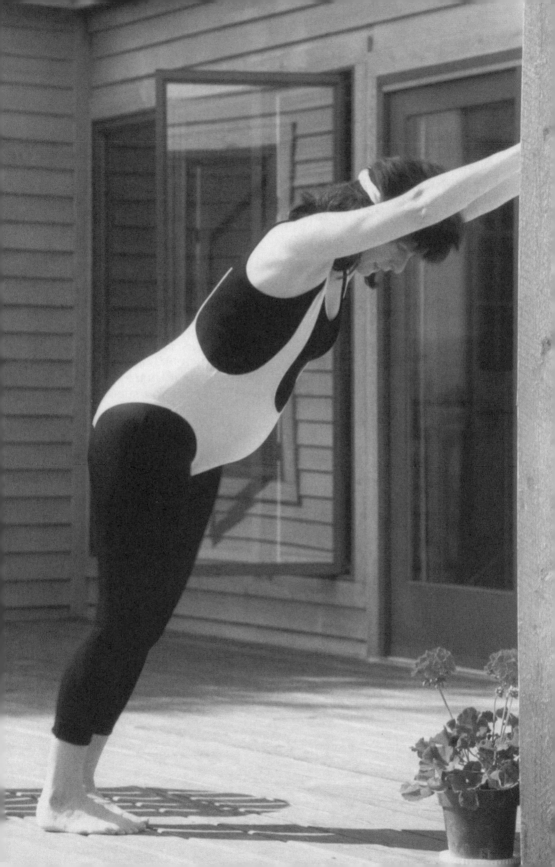

5

Keeping Active During Pregnancy

When Alpha became pregnant she was determined to keep playing tennis and doing aerobics three times a week. However, as her pregnancy progressed, the changes in her body made physical activity uncomfortable. During her sixth month, Alpha decided to take a break from physical activity. After her daughter's birth, Alpha was able to return to her pre-pregnancy level of physical activity within 6 months.

Michelle has always enjoyed walking and hoped to continue her daily 4-mile walks during pregnancy. But by her third trimester, Michelle found that her usual walks were too tiring. Because she realized that her physical activity played a big role in reducing the stress of her job, Michelle continued to walk every day, although in her ninth month she walked only a mile or two.

Say you've recently discovered the joys of exercise (or maybe you've always been a believer), but now you're pregnant. You're not sure whether to stop, slow down, or make other changes in your level of physical activity. If you are pregnant, or contemplating motherhood, you'll naturally have questions about your own exercise program. Is it safe? How will it affect you? How will it affect your baby?

Women regularly call Melpomene seeking information about the effects, beneficial or harmful, of exercise during pregnancy. While health-care providers have become more knowledgeable in the past decade, we still hear from women who have been told to cut back or quit exercising completely. An ultramarathoner calls to say, "I'm 2 months pregnant and my doctor has told me that running pounds the baby, so I stopped running. But I'm bored! Can't I run just a little?"

We continue to receive letters from women who have concerns and questions about possible negative effects of high activity levels during pregnancy. Some have questions about miscarriages; others question the conservative guidelines set forth by the American College of Obstetrics and Gynecology in 1984 for exercise during pregnancy. One aerobics instructor is "tired of hearing about a maximum heart rate of 140 when you're pregnant. I want to know how exercising at my level works with pregnancy!" She'll be glad to know those target heart rates have disappeared from the 1994 ACOG guidelines. As we have learned more about exercise and pregnancy, the experts agree that women who are very active pre-pregnancy can do more than those who are not. Recommendations should be tailored to the individual.

WHAT THE RESEARCH SAYS

Whereas in the past women were usually told to stop exercising completely during pregnancy, many health-care providers now realize that exercise can be an important adjunct to a healthy pregnancy and encourage women to be physically active. At the same time, research does not offer a clear picture of what level of exercise is really too dangerous and how this really affects the fetus.

We are not, of course, the first generation of women who have been concerned about the effects of physical labor and activity on the outcome of our pregnancies. Women throughout the world have been active during pregnancy. One of the earliest documents making reference to pregnancy and activity is the Old Testament. Exodus 1:19 states: "Hebrew women are not like Egyptian women; they are vigorous and give birth before the midwives arrive."

More recent historical references are full of both admonitions and warnings about exercising during pregnancy. An 1888 treatise entitled *Wife and Mother, or, Information for Every Woman*, coauthored by a male and a female physician, notes, "Exercise, fresh air, and occupation are then essentially necessary in pregnancy. If they be neglected, hard and tedious labors are likely to ensue." On the other hand, the same authors warn, "Stooping, lifting of heavy weights, and over-reaching ought to be carefully avoided. Running, horse-back riding, and dancing are likewise dangerous—they frequently induce a miscarriage."

Do we have any better advice today than we had in 1888? Do we know more than the people of biblical times? In a Melpomene study of pregnant runners and swimmers, more than 90 percent of these

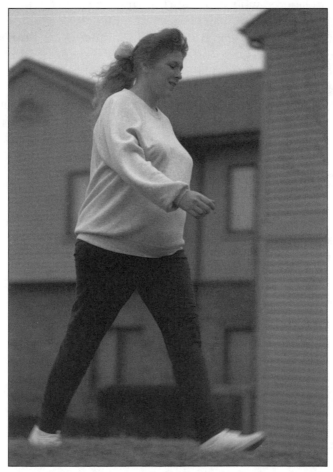

Many pregnant women say that they continue their exercise routine with their health-care provider's blessing.

women said that their health-care provider was supportive of their desire to exercise while pregnant. In a comparable group of non-exercising pregnant women, however, only 60 percent said their health-care provider made positive comments about exercise and pregnancy. Neither group of professionals were able to fully answer questions about exercise and pregnancy, nor could they supply specific information. About 75 percent of the exercising pregnant women believed their providers to be knowledgeable about the issue.

Research Limitations

Why is research information rarely available? Clearly, ethical questions must be considered when studying humans. First, only limited research can be conducted on human beings. A pregnant woman, for instance, cannot remain in a research lab for 9 months to be studied under controlled conditions. Second, it would not be ethical to knowingly cause a mother to overexert herself so that possible effects on the baby could be measured.

As a result the medical community is forced to turn to animal studies for answers. While they may provide the best information possible, animals are not women! And while new studies, using both animals and women as subjects, have been completed since the first edition of *The Bodywise Woman* in 1990, much of the research has used samples that are either too small or restrictive. In addition, different types of exercise produce different results. Therefore, researchers cannot make a definitive statement in looking at the effect of physical activity on pregnancy. Finally, the outcome of pregnancy will be based on many factors, of which exercise is only one.

Melpomene's Findings

This lack of information prompted Melpomene in 1983 to initiate a descriptive study of pregnant, exercising women in a natural, rather than a laboratory, setting. We asked 77 runners and 27 swimmers to complete a series of questionnaires during their term. They recorded their medical histories, patterns of exercise, nutrition, discomfort, and finally, their labor and delivery experiences. We also followed a group of 27 non-exercising women so we could compare their experiences during pregnancy, labor, and delivery with those of the exercising women. At 2 months and 6 months after their babies were born we checked up on each woman's health and exercise patterns as well as her child's health and development.

Here are some of the results:

1. The women who exercised did not experience any more miscarriages or infant deaths than the general population.
2. Twenty-two percent of the women who exercised had cesarean sections, which is comparable to the general population.
3. The women who exercised gained less weight than the women who did not exercise. On the average, runners gained 25 pounds, swimmers gained 27 pounds, and non-exercising women gained 31 pounds.
4. Labors were similar for all three groups.
5. The average weights of all the infants were in the normal range. On the average, babies born to swimmers weighed 7 pounds, 2 ounces; those of runners weighed 7 pounds, 9 ounces; and those of non-exercising women weighed 7 pounds, 14 ounces.
6. APGAR scores, a measure of newborn well-being, were similar for all groups.
7. The main benefits of exercising during pregnancy were psychological. As one woman wrote, "Exercise gives me an alive feeling—pregnancy is a natural state; you are limited, but by no means incapable. My spirits soared as I walked and dreamed and talked to our baby. You get more oxygen and so does the baby. Inactivity causes a vicious cycle of fatigue."
8. Runners decreased both their mileage and pace as their pregnancies progressed. Their average mileage per week in the first trimester was 21.2 miles at a pace of 8.87 minutes per mile. In the third trimester their average mileage was 7.5 miles per week at a pace of 10.68 minutes per mile.
9. Forty-one of the 77 runners continued to run into the third trimester. Only two swimmers stopped before the third trimester, one because of a sinus infection and the other because she was bothered by dry skin.
10. The majority of the women in the study felt exercise to be beneficial during pregnancy, even if they were not exercising regularly.

What we learned from these women, and from a previous Melpomene study of 195 women who ran during their pregnancies, is consistent with most other studies of the natural histories of women exercising during pregnancy. For the most part, women and their babies tolerate physical activity very well. From a psychological standpoint, exercising women said being physically active was definitely an emotional plus.

Additional Advice

Research by Dr. James Clapp has put to rest fears that exercise might negatively influence fetal weight gain. In a 1984 study, Clapp found that women who exercised aerobically in the third trimester had lower maternal weight gains, shorter gestational lengths, and fetal birth weights about a pound less than women who did not exercise, or who stopped exercising before 28 weeks. This finding concerned researchers because babies with lower birth weights may be subject to health and developmental problems, although that was not the case in Clapp's study, where both mothers and babies remained healthy. Clapp's continued research in this area documented that reduction in birth weight averaged 300-500 grams and was mainly the result of less subcutaneous fat in newborns. It's also important to note that heavier, fatter babies are not necessarily healthier. In addition, Clapp found that in fit mothers who continued to exercise during pregnancy, there was no increase in spontaneous abortion.

In February 1994, the American College of Obstetrics and Gynecology published an updated educational guide for obstetrician-gynecologists that states, "There are no data in humans to indicate that pregnant women should limit exercise intensity and lower target heart rates because of potential adverse effects." Some restrictions may cause women to cut back or stop exercising, but in general there have been no proven problems with exercising during pregnancy.

Of course, this does not mean that "anything goes" during pregnancy. For example, a 1978 survey (the most recent in the literature) of 208 scuba divers suggests babies born to women who continue to dive during pregnancy have a high number of birth defects. Pressure, chilling, and a combination of other factors may have dangerous implications for pregnant scuba divers. Therefore, the official position of the Underseas Medical Society discourages women from diving during pregnancy until further studies are completed.

While new information has become available that further supports a woman's decision to remain active during pregnancy, most women have many questions. In this chapter, we will review what is known about some of the specific issues, including cardiovascular and respiratory system responses of both mother and fetus, maternal musculoskeletal effects, thermoregulatory concerns, nutritional needs, labor and delivery experiences, and postpartum considerations.

In reviewing the available data, remember that there will always be limits to what we know. We have already mentioned the technical and ethical limits to what research can be done. In addition, what happens during a pregnancy is influenced by many personal variables, such as

An Iron Family Portrait

Barb Bradley's experience is the exception rather than the average. We've included her story here so that the truly elite athlete can see how Barb adjusted her training during pregnancy.

By the time he was born, after 33 hours of labor, Blaine Bradley Limberg had completed four triathlons, a biathlon, and a cross–country ski race. One of the triathlons included the World Championship Hawaii Ironman, a grueling event for anyone, which includes a 2-mile ocean swim, a 110-mile bike ride, and a marathon run (26.2 miles). Blaine's mom, Barb, completed the Ironman when she was 3-1/2 months pregnant. As soon as her pregnancy was confirmed, she wondered if she could still compete in the Ironman without risk to her child. After consulting the midwives and ob/gyn managing her pregnancy as well as others who had information about exercise and pregnancy, Barb decided to be especially careful in three areas:

1. Temperature. She wanted to keep her core temperature below 101 degrees F.
2. Fluids. Urinating every 2 to 3 hours was Barb's way of being sure she was taking in enough fluids.
3. Fatigue. One of the actions Barb took to avoid fatigue was to cut back her training by about half. She says this was a personal, subjective decision and not based on any specific recommendations.

Overall, Barb had an easy pregnancy. She remembers that she did feel as if she were "training at altitude" and experienced some shortness of breath and fatigue. The training was generally successful, and she entered the Ironman with the attitude "I'm not a competitor. I'm a participant." As she stood on the starting line, she felt cautious, yet confident. Before her pregnancy, Barb's goal had been to complete the Ironman in 12 hours. By taking it easy, she was able to finish in 14.5 hours, yet she never pushed herself beyond what was comfortable for her or her baby. Her postrace ultrasound showed that all was well. Wisely, Barb does not want her experience used to push women to exercise during pregnancy, but she does want other women to know what can be done.

lifestyle and genetics, that cannot be factored into "averages." Pregnancy is different for each woman, depending on who we are, what we choose to do, and a certain amount of luck, good or bad. That's why paying attention to your own body will become so important.

HEART AND LUNG CONSIDERATIONS

The table below shows how your body changes physiologically when you are pregnant. Of the many anatomic and functional changes that will occur in your body during pregnancy, those in your cardiovascular and respiratory systems will show up most strikingly when you begin to exercise.

Physiological Changes During Pregnancy

Parameter	Percent increase	Percent decrease	Unchanged
Respiratory system			
Tidal volume	30-40		
Respiratory rate			X
Resistance of tracheobronchial tree		36	
Expiratory reserve		40	
Residual volume		40	
Functional residual capacity		25	
Vital capacity			X
Respiratory minute volume	40		
Cardiovascular system			
Heart			
Rate	0-20		
Stroke volume	X		
Cardiac output	20-30		
Blood pressure			X
Peripheral blood flow	600		
Blood volume	48		
Blood constituents			
Leukocytes	70-100		
Fibrinogen	50		
Platelets	33		
Carbon dioxide		25	
Standard bicarbonate		10	
Proteins		15	

(continued)

Physiological Changes During Pregnancy (cont.)

Parameter	Percent increase	Percent decrease	Unchanged
Cardiovascular system (continued)			
Blood constituents (continued)			
Lipids	33		
Phospholipids	30-40		
Cholesterol	100		
Clotting factors I, VII, VIII, IX, X, XIII	X	X	
Gastrointestinal system			
Cardiac sphincter tone		X	
Acid secretion		X	
Motility		X	
Gallbladder emptying		X	
Urinary tract			
Renal plasma flow	25-50		
Glomerular filtration rate	50		
Ureter tone		X	
Ureteral motility			X
Metabolism			
Nitrogen stores	X		
General stores of			
Sodium	X		
Potassium	X		
Calcium	X		
Oxygen consumption	14		

Reprinted, with permission, from E.J. Quilligan and I.H. Kaiser, 1977, "Maternal Physiology." In *Obstetrics and Gynecology*, 3rd ed., edited by D.N. Danforth (Philadelphia: Harper and Row), 282.

Increasing Demands of Exercise and Pregnancy

Your heart and lungs must work overtime to meet the increased energy needs of pregnancy. Your baby is growing, your own tissues are increasing, and more blood is being pumped through your body as a result of an increase in heart rate. Blood volume, the total amount of blood in your body, also increases.

Contrary to what many women think, you don't lose your fitness level during pregnancy. In fact, your oxygen consumption—a measure of fitness that is also called aerobic capacity—increases throughout your term until it is 30 percent greater than the nonpregnant level.

Studies indicate that you can actually increase this aerobic capacity by exercising while you are pregnant. Some runners talk about the "training effect" of pregnancy due to the increased load. You may feel different when you exercise, however, because you're carrying more weight and it takes more energy to do the same activities you did before you were pregnant. Exercise physiologists describe this by saying activities have a higher "energy cost" during pregnancy. Some women see pregnancy as a challenge to continue their exercise program despite the increased "energy cost." In the later stages of pregnancy, however, fatigue and additional weight can become more problematic. Switching to non-weight-bearing exercise such as swimming may also make exercising more comfortable as the pregnancy progresses. One runner recommends, "Slow down. Don't set yourself up to do the impossible. Give yourself a time to be less compulsive."

Blood Flow to Fetus

You may also hyperventilate or feel breathless during pregnancy, which can be a drawback when you exercise. One runner told us, "For me, the first month was the hardest because my breathing was much more strained. Once I got used to it, the running was easier." Some of this breathlessness occurs because you are more sensitive to carbon dioxide, an effect stimulated by the increased progesterone (a hormone) in your body. Also, as your uterus grows, it pushes up against your diaphragm. In response, your lower ribs flare and your chest expands in an attempt to preserve lung capacity. This makes it more difficult to get a deep breath.

In this and many other ways, the female body is adapted to handle the extra energy load associated with being pregnant. What happens, then, when we add the demands of exercise to this load? Can our hearts and lungs meet this increased demand? When we exercise, our bodies deal with stress by diverting some blood flow away from the internal tissues and toward the muscles that are doing the work. Since blood is the vehicle that carries oxygen to the fetus, researchers wonder whether strenuous exercise might divert some oxygen-filled blood away from the fetus, resulting in fetal hypoxia, or lack of oxygen.

Since fetuses have undeveloped lungs, gas exchange (oxygen and carbon dioxide) occurs at the placenta instead of the lungs. Therefore, less blood reaching the placenta could theoretically result in less oxygen (carried in the blood) available for the fetus. However, animal studies have shown that fetuses are not affected unless at least 50 percent of uterine blood flow is redistributed. In addition, according to Dr. Pat Kulpa, "Rhythmic exercise should aid venous return to the heart, whereas static (isometric) forms of exercise may accentuate the venous flow problem." Therefore, the movement of exercise may help to keep the blood flowing instead of pooling in one region.

We are now able to observe blood flow to the uterus and fetus using Doppler waveforms. However, these observations yield conflicting results. Some researchers have looked at how the fetus's heart rate changes as a result of the mother's exercise. They suspect that this may tell us, indirectly, how much blood flow, and therefore oxygen, is reaching the fetus. According to a 1994 *Journal of the American College of Sports Medicine* report, maternal exercise causes a 10- to 30-beats-per-minute increase in fetal heart rate which returns to normal after about 15-30 minutes. In addition, the *Journal* reports, "No mortality or morbidity has *ever* been linked to exercise induced fetal heart rate changes in women with normal pregnancies."

We still do not know how repeated, prolonged episodes of high-intensity maternal exercise might influence fetal development. Ethical considerations keep us from studying the effects of long-term, high-intensity exercise in the lab, but the body's own defenses may prevent women from engaging in this kind of activity anyway. After a while, very strenuous activity becomes quite uncomfortable for pregnant women, especially later in their term. Perhaps these discomforts are a natural safety valve—your body's way of forcing you to cut back on activity. Pregnant women themselves have commented about their voluntary change in exercise habits.

"I've been physically active all my life," says Linda. "I expected to have an active pregnancy. Until I was 7-1/2 months pregnant I walked and cross-country skied without any problems or discomfort. But one day I noticed that my baby's position had shifted. All of a sudden it was really uncomfortable to walk." Linda had also been swimming throughout her pregnancy, and that became her exercise of choice. "Swimming remained very comfortable; it helped me relax. My body let me know when to make changes."

MUSCLE AND BONE EFFECTS

No research on exercise and pregnancy has yet been done by orthopedists or physical therapists who work most directly with the musculoskeletal system. The major concerns for physically active women in this area are back pain, hip pain, and a loosening of the joints associated with pregnancy.

Posture and Back Pain

During pregnancy, your center of gravity moves forward and upward as your baby grows and your breasts enlarge. To compensate for these changes, many women slump their shoulders and arch their backs. The resulting back curvature, called lumbar lordosis, can cause fatigue and lower back pain. About 50 percent of pregnant women experience this kind of back pain. Whether or not your back will hurt seems to have nothing to do with how much weight you gain or how much your baby weighs. However, there does seem to be an increase in back pain with increasing maternal age and number of previous pregnancies.

Some obstetricians tell us they are referring more women to physical therapists. "Many of my patients tell me they are very successful in helping minimize the pain," reports Dr. Susan Cushman, cofounder of Melpomene.

We do not know for sure what role exercise plays in back problems during pregnancy. We do know that abdominal muscles help support the back as well as the uterus. Therefore, developing good abdominal muscle tone going into pregnancy may be one way to lessen backache problems. Also, according to Dr. Raul Artal and colleagues in 1990, "Low back pain may be reduced by improving strength, endurance, and control of the muscles attached to the spine and pelvis." In cases of severe back pain, though, exercise can actually be harmful. It is best to check with your health-care provider before exercising with considerable back pain.

Another consideration that will become more obvious as your pregnancy progresses is a change in balance caused by increased weight and a shift in your center of gravity. If you participate in sports requiring great balance and agility, you'll need to be aware that these changes may affect your ability to perform at pre-pregnancy levels. A physician working with downhill skiers noticed that the first sign of pregnancy in one of her clients was a rapid deterioration in skiing skill that put her at greater risk for injury.

Echoing trends in the general population, half of the runners, swimmers, and non-exercising women in the Melpomene study experienced back pain during pregnancy. As with other pregnancy-related aches, pains, and physical problems, the women tried to adjust their habits to decrease these discomforts. A triathlete who participated in our research developed back pain in the second trimester, reportedly due to an uncomfortable chair at work. Since her back was particularly sore in the evenings (the only time she could exercise), she often cut back on the duration and intensity of her workout.

Another woman who ran in the Olympic marathon trials during her second trimester experienced lower back pain. She was accustomed to running 10 miles per day but said, "At about 5 months, I had lower back problems after running. I had to decrease my mileage to 3 miles or less at a time. I learned that leaning forward while I ran helped ease the pressure." It is important to let your body be your guide.

Dr. Mona Shangold, an obstetrician/gynecologist interested in sports medicine, believes that all women, including pregnant women, should be encouraged to participate in some sort of strength training program to strengthen their upper body and help avoid back problems. The originators of one maternal fitness program have tried to combine strength training with aerobic conditioning to decrease discomfort and also to prepare women for labor and delivery. In their research, they found that women who were pregnant for the first time were less likely to undergo a cesarean section if they participated regularly in this program. Average time in labor was not affected. All the women in the exercise program reported that they enjoyed it, no matter what their level of participation.

Softening Ligaments and Cartilage

The hormone relaxin, which is secreted by the ovary, and possibly the pregnant uterus and placenta, is detectable only in pregnant women. Relaxin causes the body's connective tissues, the ligaments and carti- lage, to soften and stretch so that the pelvic outlet will be able to accommodate the baby at birth. Though this softening proves to be a great help during delivery, it may subject your joints to undue strain during pregnancy. It becomes easier to turn an ankle, or twist a knee, for instance, because your joints are able to stretch farther than they normally would, and the stabilizing ligaments are more pliable. You'll want to be aware of these changes as you exercise.

The round ligaments that support your uterus become stretched as the fetus grows. Some women who engage in activities such as running, in which there can be movement that tugs these ligaments, experience pain in one or both sides of their lower abdomen. While this is uncomfortable, it is not harmful to either you or your baby. Women who do not exercise also experience round ligament pain during normal daily activities. Some Melpomene members have reported that an elastic abdominal support, stretchy running/ biking shorts, or a tank-type swimsuit eliminates or relieves the problem.

**Elastic Maternity Belt
for Adominal Support**

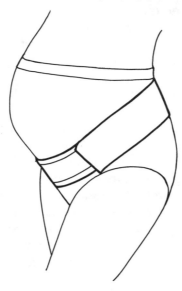

Unlike muscle fiber, which is elastic, connective tissue does not regain its shape once it is stretched. Your abdominal muscles are joined in the middle by a vertical band of connective tissue called the linea alba. Many pregnant women experience a separation of this seam, a condition known as diastasis recti.

Early in pregnancy, abdominal tone can be maintained with crunches or curls. During the last trimester the size of the uterus usually prevents exercises that use the abdominal muscles. Moderate straight leg lifts may still be possible and will not cause problems.

If you are aware of these muscle and skeletal changes that occur during pregnancy, you can modify your exercise patterns to accommodate these changes safely. Strengthening your upper body and the abdominal muscles, and practicing good posture can be done before pregnancy and can help prevent, or alleviate, your discomforts in the coming months.

Overheating

Most recommendations and guidelines about exercise during pregnancy warn against overheating. At Melpomene, we advise pregnant women to avoid exercising in hot and/or humid environments and to be sure to drink enough fluids. The reasons for these recommendations are understandable if we consider the mechanisms for thermoregulation.

Your body has ingenious ways of getting rid of the heat you naturally generate. The heat is conducted outward to your skin and is dissipated as blood runs through the capillaries close to the surface. Your sweat glands provide a water-based cooling system. As sweat on your skin evaporates, it gives up heat, making you feel cooler in the process. During pregnancy heat is generated both by you and by the fetus. More blood is pumped to the skin, and more sweat is produced by the sweat glands. Sometimes, when the air outside the body is hot and humid, this cooling system can't work as efficiently, and both you and the fetus can become overheated.

Numerous researchers, including Mottola, Bell, and Dreiling, have found through animal studies that maternal overheating early in gestation can cause defects in the fetus. We can't necessarily apply these studies to humans, however, because some of the animals have cooling mechanisms such as panting that are quite different from the mechanisms we use. Thermoregulation is probably most important in humans in the first trimester because of heat-sensitive fetal developments of the major organ systems. However, there is limited data on core body temperatures during exercise for pregnant women. Nevertheless, experts are convinced that the possible dangers of overheating are something to take into consideration, especially during exercise.

Exercise and Body Temperature

Of course, your temperature is bound to rise somewhat as you exercise. Keeping it within safe limits is the key. Researchers in Pennsylvania measured the core temperatures of four pregnant women before, during, and after they ran on a treadmill. All four women were runners before becoming pregnant and still ran regularly. Their temperatures did increase during exercise and remained elevated for at least 15 minutes afterwards. Researchers noted that temperature reduction to pre-exercise levels was especially slow during the third trimester. The researchers felt, however, that the temperature increases they saw were not dangerous. All the women went on to deliver healthy babies. While this is a reassuring study, it is important to note that it involved only four women and that they were already accustomed to exercising. Their rise in temperature may not have been as great as that of an unconditioned woman. Moreover, the length of time they exercised while their temperatures were measured was only 20 minutes.

Recently other scientists compared core temperatures of pregnant women who exercised for 20 minutes on a stationary bike when the bike was on dry land and when it was in water. Although temperature rose in both mediums, it didn't rise quite as high in the women who biked in the water. Many women, in fact, choose to swim in extremely hot

Gayle Winegar: Fit for Two

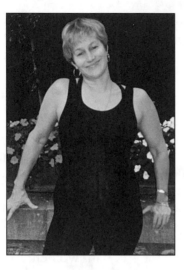

Gayle Winegar is the owner of the Sweatshop, a small, full-service health club. She became pregnant for the first time at age 40. "I've always been physically active. I started dancing when I was three. As a teenager, I was active in gymnastics, horseback riding, swimming, and running.

"I've felt I had to diet and lose weight all my life, so I was surprised at the feedback my new body got. I've never had so many people continuously telling me how great I looked. My skin, my hair—everything. Suddenly my weight was no longer an issue. It was the most physically freeing time I've ever had. Even though I was going through all these changes, it was all for the cause of having a baby. Suddenly, even though my breasts were getting big and my belly was hanging out, it was all wonderful. I think pregnancy is the first time that you feel the true purposes for your breasts and hips. You realize, 'Hey these aren't here just for show.'

"I wore leotards throughout my pregnancy. Maternity clothes look like you're trying to hide things, like 'shame on me, I had sex. I better live under a tent.' One day I walked into a maternity shop wearing a short leopard-skin minidress, so my belly really hung out—kind of risqué for pregnancy, and I thought I might raise some eyebrows. But the woman at the shop told me that in Europe even the maternity clothes are tight-fitting. What does that tell you about the American psyche? Here we see women as sex symbols if they are thin and tall and leggy. The European notion of what a woman is is so much broader."

Gayle taught aerobics classes until three weeks before she delivered the "perfect baby." "It felt so good to move. I was in great shape when I got pregnant, working out and eating well. I had so much energy to work! If I could have stayed at the second trimester hormonal level forever, my business would have just boomed."

Now that she's a mom, Gayle is finding a few problems she didn't anticipate. "For one thing, time is a big issue. I haven't had the time to work out since my baby was born. I'm still trying to figure out how to both be a mom and run a business!"

weather just because it is more comfortable than land exercise. Exercising in normal temperature water (~83 degrees F) may be superior to land because of the smaller increase in maternal core body temperature, according to the *Journal of the American College of Sports Medicine.*

A study by James Clapp and Raul Artal found that there were no demonstrated neural tube or other defects among pregnant women who performed even vigorous exercise. This is significant because the neural tube becomes the spinal cord. Its formation is one of the most heat-sensitive processes during fetal development. In another Clapp study, the peak temperatures declined over time for pregnant, exercising women. He concluded that women may physiologically adapt to pregnancy.

Hot Tubs and Saunas

Some women wonder about the safety of hot tubs and saunas during pregnancy. Researchers who studied the medical histories of women with children who had birth defects did find a connection between raised temperatures and birth defects. In these cases, the mothers either had prolonged fevers during early pregnancy, or had spent long periods of time in hot tubs or saunas. These kinds of congenital problems are rare in Finland, however, where nearly everyone takes saunas. A survey of the sauna habits of 100 pregnant Finnish women found that women who took saunas before pregnancy continued to do so when pregnant. There was a trend over the course of the 9 months of pregnancy to shorten the length of time in the sauna and to lower the temperature of the sauna. In this instance, common sense led women to protect themselves. American obstetricians get many more questions regarding hot tubs, which are much more popular in the U.S. than saunas. Their recommendation is to stay in the hot tubs at a temperature that seems comfortable and for only a short time.

How to Avoid Overheating

So, what can an expectant mother do to avoid overheating?
1. Don't exercise in hot, humid environments. Sometimes an air-conditioned health club or a pool may be the best way to beat the heat.
2. Drink more fluids. The more fluids you have, the more freely you will perspire, and the cooler you'll be. Drinking enough fluids is also important to avoid dehydration, which has also been associated with premature labor.
3. Stop exercising if you are too warm. As with many other activities during pregnancy, comfort is the key. There is no reason to

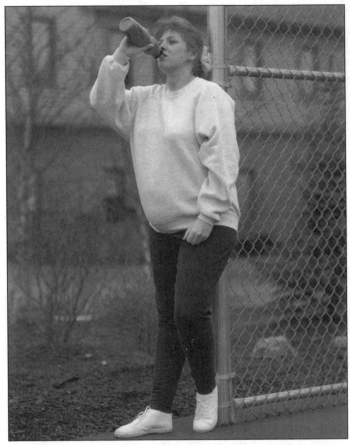

Drink plenty of fluids to keep from overheating during exercise.

subject yourself to any risk, no matter how minimal, by overheating. A shorter, less intense workout may be a wise choice
on warm days. Everyone who exercises tries to minimize heat
stress, and pregnant women should be even more careful.

4. Keep the hot tub at a temperature that feels comfortable, and
stay in for only a short time. This may be far below your normal
level of comfort, especially as your pregnancy progresses.

DIETARY AND HEALTH CONCERNS DURING PREGNANCY

When women in the Melpomene study of exercise during pregnancy
were asked if they had made any changes in their health habits during

their pregnancies, the majority indicated they were trying to improve their dietary and eating patterns. Some were eating more protein. Many had increased the amounts of calcium-rich dairy products they ate. Others had cut out junk foods.

No research has been done on the nutritional requirements of physically active pregnant or breast-feeding women. According to Janet King, PhD in nutrition, we can only draw inferences from what we know about pregnant, sedentary women and nonpregnant, active women. We do know, for instance, that a woman's nutritional habits before and during pregnancy (and afterwards if she is breast-feeding) are important for the health of the mother and child. The mother's weight gain will affect the weight of the baby at birth. Birth weights are important because preterm and growth-retarded babies are often at risk for health and developmental problems.

Another concern during pregnancy is gestational diabetes. It's important to note that regular exercise may help prevent the development of this condition. Nutritionist Marion Franz and her associates at the International Diabetes Center believe that exercise is also important for diabetic women as well as women at risk for diabetes because it can help keep blood glucose at more normal levels. They recommend taking a walk after eating, when blood sugars tend to be elevated. If you are aware of a condition such as this in your own medical history, you may want to contact an association that distributes information and conducts research on the condition. Ask your health-care provider where to find these resources.

What About Weight Gain During Pregnancy?

Until the early 1970s women were advised to limit weight gain to 20 pounds or less. The main concern was toxemia (also called preeclampsia). Toxemia is a general term used to describe a serious disorder of pregnancy in which hypertension, protein in the urine, and edema (fluid retention) occur. Experts mistakenly believed that weight gain caused toxemia, when in reality it was the other way around. Toxemia caused the weight gain through fluid retention. At the same time, scientists developed the theory that the fetus is a perfect parasite whose nutritional needs would always be met from the mother's stores or intake. Thus, women began to restrict their diets to prevent toxemia, thinking that the fetus would just naturally adjust to the lower food intake.

Today, although we know better, women are still restricting their diets, this time for different reasons. The myth that says women have to be thin to be attractive is alive and well, and larger women, pregnant

Suggested Weight Gain

Underweight women (BMI<19.8): 28-40 pounds at 40 weeks with a gain of 2 pounds per week during second and third trimesters

Normal-weight women (BMI19.8-26.0): 25-35 pounds at 40 weeks with a gain of 1 pound per week during second and third trimesters

Overweight women (BMI>26): 15-25 pounds at 40 weeks with a gain of .5 to .75 pound per week during second and third trimesters

Data from Agostini 1994.

or not, are seen as lacking in self-control. Despite the fact that it can be detrimental to mother and baby, a few women still put themselves on a strict diet throughout their pregnancy. Many women feel anxious about the weight they gain when pregnant, even if it's a normal, healthy amount; however, pregnancy is not the time to restrict your diet. Therefore, women who come into a pregnancy with an eating disorder should be aware of the negative effects of disordered eating on the developing fetus. Dr. Susan Cushman, who has a large obstetric practice, reports, however, that most women with eating disorders have been able to improve their eating habits during pregnancy.

Many women who have always considered themselves sensible eaters are less sure about what to do during pregnancy. We can offer some basic guidelines. There is no such thing as a "best" weight gain during pregnancy. In general a 20- to 40-pound weight gain is appropriate for most women. Factors to be considered include your pre-pregnancy weight and your level of physical activity. If you are thin, you may need to gain more than a heavier woman. If you are physically active, you'll need to eat enough to cover the cost of fetal growth, added maternal tissue, and the energy needed for physical activity.

Keep in mind that most women lose 15 pounds with the actual birth and another 5 pounds over the first week. While you certainly want to eat enough for yourself and your baby, a 50- to 60-pound weight gain will take much longer to lose.

Eating Enough of the Right Foods

Of course, when you're interested in good nutrition, it's not only the quantity of food taken in (the total number of calories) that is important, but also the quality of the diet. Research shows that some pregnant women can gain weight even at normal intake levels. The mechanism for this is not known. It may be that a pregnant woman's metabolism becomes more efficient. It may also be that pregnant women instinctively decrease their level of activity and therefore save energy. Many women will gain an appropriate amount of weight in pregnancy without changing their normal eating habits.

The body also seems to be well adapted to make the most of what you feed it during pregnancy. But again, the question arises, "What if you add exercise to the equation? Will that change your nutritional needs?" In Melpomene Institute studies on the nutritional habits of physically active women based on diet histories and activity logs, pregnant runners consumed fewer calories than what would normally be required by their level of physical activity. Yet, these women were gaining weight appropriately, perhaps through some of the mechanisms mentioned here.

Why You Might Experience Appetite Changes

Keep in mind that pregnancy itself may change your eating habits, especially when physical changes begin to affect your appetite. For example, morning sickness early in pregnancy, which may be due to high levels of human chorionic gonadotropic hormone (HCG), will make crackers look more attractive than steak. Frequent small snacks may agree better with you than three larger meals. For those women who want to continue to exercise, changing workouts to afternoon or evening can eliminate unpleasant or impossible morning workouts.

Some of the unpleasant side effects of pregnancy, such as nausea, heartburn, indigestion, and constipation, are caused by an increase in a steroid called progesterone. Progesterone causes the smooth muscles of the gastrointestinal tract to relax so that food moves through the stomach and bowels more slowly, leaving you with the feeling of fullness, heartburn, or nausea. Slower movement in the gut also means that more water is absorbed by the intestines—a probable cause of constipation. Exercise is often recommended as a way to promote regu–larity, and the pregnant women in our study vouched for its effectiveness.

Progesterone is also responsible for an increase in appetite felt by pregnant women. (Yes, it's true: You really might feel hungrier when you are pregnant!) But as pregnancy progresses and your uterus begins to displace your other internal organs, you may prefer to eat several small meals rather than a few large meals.

The Need for Increased Nutrients

New research has documented the importance of folic acid in a healthy pregnancy. Women planning or hoping to become pregnant should take a folic acid supplement of .5 to 1 milligram per day to reduce the risk of some birth defects. You should continue to take folic acid during the pregnancy. This supplement may be obtained either through a prescription or in the form of an over-the-counter prenatal vitamin. Pregnant women should also be aware of the increased need for iron and calcium. Anemia is common in pregnancy because there is an increase in blood volume (the liquid portion of blood) with a lesser rise in red blood cells. Most health-care providers prescribe a prenatal vitamin containing iron for pregnant women, since most do not get enough iron in the foods they eat. This is not true of calcium; it appears that metabolic and physiologic changes help the body actually conserve calcium during pregnancy. In general, for women who were getting enough calcium in their pre-pregnancy diets, supplements during pregnancy did not seem to make much difference. However, diet logs from the Melpomene studies of pregnant exercisers indicate that most women did not meet RDA for all necessary nutrients, including iron, in their normal diets. Taking a prenatal vitamin is recommended for most pregnant women to help ensure that nutritional needs are being met. We do not yet have enough information to know whether there are additional specific nutrient needs for pregnant women who exercise. To be on the safe side, you'd be wise to make sure your diet is high in vitamins and minerals. Whether you are pregnant or not, dietary supplements do not take the place of a good diet.

GUIDELINES FOR EXERCISE DURING PREGNANCY

"Stay within your body's limits—it will 'tell' you to back off if problems arise."

Michele Davis, a nationally ranked woman runner who ran in the Olympic marathon trial during one of her two "running" pregnancies.

Some animal research and the experience of pregnant women who exercise suggest that exercising within your comfort range is the best general guideline. Pregnant woman can expect more support from doctors and midwives than was true even in the 1980s because these practitioners have had more experience with pregnant women who exercise. Health-care providers are more likely to encourage exercise because they have now followed many successful exercising pregnancies. Says Dr. Susan Cushman, "Most of us would love to get our patients off the couch." Gynecologists received their first set of guidelines from the American College of Obstetrics and Gynecology in 1985. These recommended a maximum heart rate of 140 beats per minute. Many women and some physicians believed it was too conservative. Fit women felt that they could not get a good workout at such a low rate. The 1994 guidelines are more liberal and do not include the previous heart rate maximum.

We at Melpomene believe that the 1994 guidelines more closely mirror our recommendations for pregnant women that appeared in our journal and the first edition of *The Bodywise Woman*. Our recommendations are based specifically on the research we have done coupled with commonsense tips and knowledge provided by obstetricians with years of practice and experience. Remember that for many sports, only anecdotal reports and little or no direct research data are available from which to develop guidelines. Because we have worked primarily with pregnant runners and swimmers and with maternal fitness programs, we offer a separate list of more specific guidelines for these activities.

We'll begin with general guidelines for anyone considering exercise while pregnant. Beyond this, we strongly encourage each individual to seek out guidelines that speak to your own situation.

For women who have not exercised regularly prior to pregnancy, doctors and midwives hold a variety of opinions on whether pregnancy is a good time to begin a serious exercise program. Melpomene frequently hears from women who are ready or anxious to make lifestyle changes and want to know more about the role of exercise in pregnancy. In general, we suggest that women in good health can begin an exercise program after checking with their health-care provider.

General Guidelines

1. Discuss your exercise plans with your health-care provider, especially if medical conditions might present problems such as threatened preterm labor, placenta previa, or a twin pregnancy.
2. Talk over your desire to be physically active with people who are important to you. Their psychological support can be very

helpful. Ignore comments or advice from people who are not important to you.

3. Listen to your body. "No pain, no gain" does not apply to exercising during pregnancy.

4. Wear comfortable clothing. Buy cushioned, stable shoes, a good bra, and shorts that are not constricting. Most women find tank-type swimming suits best.

5. Be flexible. Do not have preset goals for exercising during pregnancy. Be prepared to stop or switch to another form of exercise if you experience persistent discomfort or are chronically fatigued.

6. Avoid an anaerobic (breathless) pace. Your ability to perform will vary depending on pre-pregnancy patterns and the level of fitness you maintain during pregnancy. Expect gradual decreases from pre-pregnancy competitive fitness.

7. Exercise within your comfort range. Exercising to the point of exhaustion, or feeling chronically fatigued, is detrimental to both mother and fetus.

8. Learn all you can about exercising during pregnancy in order to have examples of how much discomfort is "ordinary" and what may be reason for concern.

9. Avoid overheating and dehydration. Drink plenty of fluids before, during, and after your exercise routine.

10. Minimize the risk of injury to joints and ligaments. Take the time to adequately warm up and cool down. Avoid stretching to the point of maximum resistance. Pay attention to your balance and posture.

11. Be sure to meet your nutritional needs. A healthy weight gain is a good indicator that you are eating enough.

12. Once you start, stay in the habit of exercising. Exercise 20 to 60 minutes, three to five times a week, preferably on alternate days. Irregular or infrequent exercise can lead to injury and fatigue.

How to Evaluate Maternal Fitness Programs

Maternal fitness programs have become quite popular in recent years, and there are a number of classes to choose from, including some on videocassette. Although no thorough, independent evaluation of any of these programs has been done, we can offer you some help in selecting a program that will be safe and effective for you.

Before you begin a maternal fitness program, we suggest you consult your doctor or midwife. Discuss your exercise needs in light of your medical history and your current physical condition. Get medical approval before you begin. Then select a sound exercise program with a qualified instructor. *Be choosy.*

At the heart of a good exercise program is a well-qualified instructor. This is true whether you are attending a class or using a video. Look for an instructor who:

- is sensitive to the health education needs of pregnant women;
- has an extensive background as an exercise instructor;
- has training that includes information specific to pregnancy and childbirth;
- will assess and monitor your health fitness level, modifying the exercise program to reflect your needs; and
- will teach you:
  —to identify signs and symptoms of potential problems;
  —ways to reduce the risk of injury; and
  —the importance of fluid replacement.

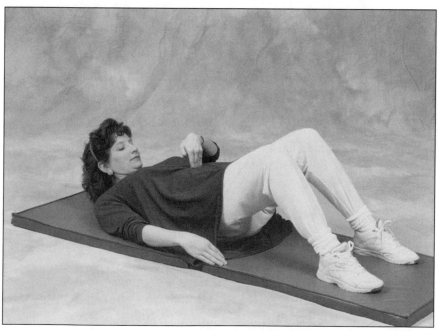

Before every exercise session that will involve your abdominals, be sure to check for separation of your abdominal muscles. If the separation is more than one inch, you'll need to take care not to strain the muscles.

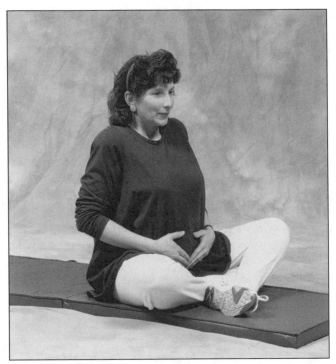

Breathe deep and easy—relaxation and breathing exercises are best done at the end of your workout, when your muscles are slightly fatigued.

In addition to a well-qualified instructor, a good prenatal exercise program will have the following basic components:

1. *Warm-up period* to protect joints and muscles from injury and to slowly increase breathing and heart rates.
2. *Muscle strengthening exercises* to build and maintain tone and strength.
3. *Cardiovascular conditioning exercises* to build and maintain heart and lung strength and endurance.
4. *Cool-down period* to safely ease breathing and heart rates to a lower level of activity.
5. *Relaxation techniques* to identify and release muscle tension.
6. *Health education and discussion period* to foster a supportive atmosphere for the discussion of concerns related to pregnancy.

Once you begin, keep exercising. Regular exercise can increase your flexibility while strengthening your heart, lungs, bones, and muscles. Now that you have established an exercise habit, keep it up for life!

Recommendations for Pregnant Swimmers

Swimming is probably the safest and most relaxing physical activity during pregnancy. The swimmers in our studies reported little discomfort even at the end of their third trimester. They offer the following advice and suggestions:

> Be sure the water and air temperatures are comfortable; leave the water if you feel uncomfortably chilled or overheated. Take time to warm up.
>
> Try doing some stretching on land or in the water. Start off swimming slowly until you loosen up.
>
> Swim according to your abilities. Use moderation, and be sure to breathe properly. Avoid diving or jumping into the water feet first.
>
> Remember to drink water both before and after exercise.
>
> Swimmers need to find a comfortable suit. Some maternity suits become too heavy when wet, making swimming difficult. Experiment with different fabrics, styles, and sizes until you find something that gives you support where you need it and still lets you swim comfortably.
>
> While it's inadvisable to swim alone, you should also avoid crowded pools to minimize the risk of being kicked.
>
> If you experience contractions, leg cramps, or joint pain, be ready to stop swimming, or change your swimming style. You may need to try different strokes, kicks, or turns. Modify or stop your exercise program if you develop medical problems such as early dilation.

Precautions

We've learned that physical activity and participation in sport enhance many pregnancies. It's also true that this is not the best time to be highly competitive.

Dr. Susan Cushman, an obstetrician who ran during her own pregnancy, tells her patients that pregnancy is not a time to prove anything. She has three suggestions for her patients: Exercise at about two-thirds of your normal intensity, don't overheat, and don't let yourself become dehydrated. Some additional precautions, however, apply to specific sports.

These activities are not advised during pregnancy:

- Scuba diving (try snorkeling instead!)
- Waterskiing (danger of falling on an unstable surface and damage to internal organs from water forced intra-vaginally)
- Rock climbing (after the first trimester)
- Hang gliding
- Snowmobiling (other than low-speed, sedate touring)
- Martial arts involving throws and contact

Any physical activity or sport that has serious risks for you also puts your fetus at risk. Accidents can and do happen. Potentially risky activities include:

- Bicycling (consider the risks of a bike/car accident or a serious fall)
- Downhill or cross-country skiing
- Ice-skating

Some of these activities may be appropriate for the skilled person, but even then, consider those around you. An expert cyclist cannot control the cars around her any more than an expert skier can control the actions of other skiers. Think carefully before you engage in these activities, especially during the second half of pregnancy when the uterus is more vulnerable.

Team Sports

Avoid participating in a highly competitive team sport event. At a recreational level, sports such as softball, soccer, or volleyball are probably safe. In a highly competitive atmosphere you may not be able to think of the safety of your baby first.

Skill Sports

Activities such as bowling, golf, target shooting, and archery are almost certainly safe, especially if you are accustomed to them. Many women have reported that pregnancy actually improved their golf or bowling scores, at least for a time.

Racquet Sports

No one recommendation applies to all racquet sports. Tennis is safer than racquetball, handball, or squash. Bear in mind that whenever you are playing in a closed court, you run a higher risk of being hit in the abdomen with a hard-hit ball.

Recommendations for Pregnant Runners

When Melpomene began looking at exercise and pregnancy in the early 1980s running was a very popular activity. Since this was a relatively new phenomenon, many in the medical profession were cautious. While it is much easier to find good, specific advice today, these guidelines may be helpful.

One problem that is more likely to occur is overheating or not drinking enough. Run in the coolest part of the day and in appropriate clothing. Be sure to drink plenty of fluids before a run—even if you may have to stop for bathroom breaks more often.

Run with others, if possible. Always let people know when and where you are running. Take money along in case you need to phone someone to take you home. Take the time for adequate warm-up and cool-down before and after running.

Be willing to modify your runs' intensity, frequency, and speed. Increasing weight and fatigue may dictate shorter, slower runs, eliminating hills and speed work. Stop and walk if necessary. You may feel a need to slow down because of heat, ligament or joint pains, or Braxton-Hicks contractions (painless uterine tightenings).

Wear comfortable clothing. Well-cushioned, stable running shoes, a good bra, and comfortable shorts are important. Some women find that a lightweight maternity girdle offers support for the back and ligaments. (See the discussion on page 193.)

Be kind to your back. Pay attention to your posture and balance. You may want to experiment with posture changes that make you more stable while running.

Modify or stop your exercise program if medical problems such as unusual discomfort, early dilation, or bleeding develop.

Weight Lifting and Strength Training

Lifting maximal weights is not recommended because of risk of injury to joints and ligaments. Women who participate in weight or strength training prior to becoming pregnant usually switch to lighter weights as their pregnancy progresses.

LABOR AND DELIVERY

Various historical sources, including the Bible, imply that an active pregnancy is apt to make for an easier labor and delivery. Research data to support these suggestions are not as clear. Some researchers have suggested that female athletes might have more difficulty with labor and delivery because of their "overly" developed musculature. Others believe just the opposite.

Early researchers reported that elite, Olympic-caliber women athletes had easy deliveries with short second stages of labor and few cesarean sections. In more recent studies of women with first-time pregnancies, those who took part in strength training and aerobic maternal fitness programs also had a lower-than-average number of C-sections, but their labors were of average length. A third set of results comes from Dr. Pat Kulpa, an obstetrician/gynecologist, who studied women who were engaged in regular aerobic exercise as well as some who were not. Dr. Kulpa and her colleagues found that for first-time mothers, there was no difference in C-section rates between the exercising and non-exercising women. However, second-stage labor was shorter for women who exercised.

Another question is whether or not exercise puts women at risk for premature births. Jean-Claude Veille and his colleagues found that there is no increase in uterine activity among women who exercised at 70 percent of their maximum heart rate. Yet another study shows that physically active women were at a decreased risk of premature birth. Several studies note an increase in preterm deliveries for women who perform strenuous work and lifting. The American College of Sports Medicine therefore recommends that women "avoid heavy lifting, prolonged standing in the third trimester, and strenuous work in late gestation." In fact, these precautions are more likely to apply to your job than to your level of physical activity.

Conflicting findings about exercise, labor, and delivery reflect some of the problems in coming to uniform conclusions about possible benefits as well as problems of exercising while pregnant. It is hard to predict the course of labor because each woman's actual experience will be as individual as she is. Exercise is only one of the variables involved—genetics also plays a strong role.

POSTPARTUM CONSIDERATIONS

While researchers struggle with the question of whether or not exercise is safe during pregnancy, women continue to get pregnant and continue to exercise. After their babies are born, they wonder about resuming exercise, and about regaining their pre-pregnancy level of activity and fitness.

Recently the media have played up the post-pregnancy athletic performances of a few elite women. For example, in 1995, Sue Olsen of Burnsville, MN, ran Grandma's Marathon and 1 week later ran 63 miles in a 24-hour running event. She delivered a healthy baby 2 days later. Four months after the baby was born, she ran a 3:13 marathon, followed by posting the winning women's time of 8:50 in a 100K race. There is now talk of "the training effect of pregnancy." In an absurd leap, we have moved from wondering whether we should exercise during pregnancy to recommending pregnancy as a way to improve athletic ability. Aside from the anecdotal accounts, there is not much data to back up this kind of recommendation.

When Is It Safe to Begin Exercising?

Most women are advised to wait 3 to 6 weeks after an uncomplicated vaginal delivery before they start exercising again. In Melpomene's research, and from our conversations with physically active women, we know that many women do not want to wait this long. With this in mind, we decided to include a list of commonsense considerations for women who want to exercise during the immediate postpartum period. Look for them at the end of this section, on page 214.

In general, you'll want to keep in mind that your body has been changing throughout the 9 months of your pregnancy and that those changes aren't about to reverse themselves overnight. For example, relaxin softened your connective tissues so they could stretch to accommodate the growing fetus and the pressures of labor and delivery. One place this occurred was in the pelvic floor, where the muscles that hold together your internal organs are found. The fascia that connects these muscles stretched during pregnancy and, once stretched, will never regain its former shape. To compensate for the loss of support, you may want to work on strengthening your muscles in this area as well as others. Dr. Pat Kulpa notes that it takes about 6 weeks postpartum for abdominal wall tone to return to the pre-pregnancy state. Start out with walking and straight leg lifts before progressing to crunches and curls.

Kegel exercises are often recommended for strengthening the muscles in the pelvic floor. These exercises may also help lessen the problem of urinary incontinence that many women experience after delivery, especially during weight-bearing activities such as running and walking.

Kegel Exercises

Kegel exercises help strengthen the muscles that control urine flow. They were devised some 30 years ago by Dr. Arnold Kegel to help women with stress incontinence. They are designed to strengthen the pubococcygeus, the muscle that encircles the urethra (urinary opening) and the outside walls of the vagina.

Before you can do the exercises, you must first locate the pubococcygeus (P.C.) muscle. To do this, sit on the toilet, spread your legs apart, and try to stop the flow of urine midstream without moving your legs. The P.C. muscle is the one you use to stop the urine.

Now that you know where it is and what it feels like, you can begin the strengthening exercises.

First tighten the P.C. muscle as you did to stop the urine. Hold it for a count of three. Relax. Repeat the exercise 10 times, several times a day. Build to 25-30 repetitions about five times a day. You can do the contractions anywhere and at any time throughout the day—while driving a car, sitting at a desk, watching TV, waiting for the elevator, or lying in bed. Remember to breathe naturally while doing your Kegels. If you practice these exercises frequently, you will notice improved muscle tone within a few weeks or a few months.

Finding Time to Exercise

Finding time to exercise is a lesson in creative time-management for the new mother. If she chooses to breast-feed (as did more than 90 percent of the women in Melpomene's studies of exercise and pregnancy), there will be additional constraints in scheduling. We advise women to nurse first, then exercise to avoid the discomfort of overly full breasts. For the first few months, however, arranging child care to meet a baby's irregular schedule may be as stressful an exercise as you can manage!

Nutrition

Besides practical problems such as child care, breast-feeding women are also concerned about nutrition. While women want to eat and drink enough to maintain a good milk supply, many are eager to return to a lower weight. In our research, we found that women tend to greatly increase their exercise level in postpartum, while eating fewer calories than they did during pregnancy. Many asked us, "Is it all right to be losing weight while I'm breast-feeding? Is the baby getting all the nutrients needed for growth?" In a recent 1994 update on the subject Dr. Pat Kulpa says: "There are no good data to suggest that exercise has detrimental effects on the quality of milk or its production. However, proper nutrition, hydration, adequate rest . . . are essential to lactation." Overall, we feel that infant weight gain, not maternal weight loss, should be used as the measure of appropriate maternal diet by breast-feeding women.

Breast-feeding women lose residual pregnancy weight more slowly. Eventually, the breast-feeding women in our study did lose all the weight they had gained, but it took them 3-9 months after the birth. The women who were not breast-feeding lost it faster, but they also tended to be more active and to eat less.

Some researchers have expressed concern about the relation between breast-feeding and osteoporosis, a thinning of the bones that is a major health concern for women (see discussion on pages 261-271). The average woman in this country does not get enough calcium in her diet, and according to our research, this is also true for most women who exercise during pregnancy and while breast-feeding.

A recent study found that sedentary women who breast-fed for more than 6 months showed bone loss even though they had calcium intakes above the RDA . How might these women have fared if they had been exercising? Recent evidence points to the fact that exercise may actually increase bone mass. It will be important for researchers to explore the relationship among exercise, calcium intake, bone mass, and breast-feeding.

What About Fatigue and Depression?

Another postpartum reality for many new mothers is depression, fatigue, and a feeling of being overwhelmed by their new role. At 2 months postpartum, about half of all the women in Melpomene's pregnancy study perceived themselves to have experienced the "postpartum blues." This depression hit both the exercising and the non-exercising women. One woman recalled, "During the first week I was very tired and I couldn't stop crying." At this point, we do not know enough about the possible influence of exercise on postpartum depression. However, because exercise in general helps elevate moods, it also probably helps lessen postpartum mood problems.

When asked if they felt fully recovered, or back to "being themselves," after 2 months, only 53 percent of the runners, 60 percent of the swimmers, and 50 percent of the sedentary women answered yes. Many may still have been trying to recapture pre-pregnancy activity levels and/or weight. All but one woman in the study did report herself to be in good or excellent health. To all new mothers, we say, "Try not to be impatient. Postpartum is the rest of your life!"

Guidelines for Exercising After Your Baby Is Born

After the birth of the baby, most women are eager to resume pre-pregnancy activities, including exercise. Many come to us for guidelines or precautions. Unfortunately, we have little hard data, because very little research has been done on women who resume exercise after delivery. What we do pass along is information we have gleaned from the participants in our exercise and pregnancy research.

The first step is to discuss your exercise plan with your doctor or midwife. If you've had a cesarean section, it is especially important to consider your physician's instructions. These will directly relate to lifting, exercising the abdominal muscles, and very strenuous exercise.

Consider these points before you start exercising:

1. If you had an episiotomy, you will probably want to wait until all soreness is gone before you exercise vigorously. Being able to walk or sit comfortably is a sign you are ready for more vigorous exercise.
2. Since you cannot use tampons for about 4 weeks, you may find it more convenient to wait until bleeding has slowed.
3. If you exercise and begin to bleed heavily, you should give yourself more time to recover.
4. Since your hormonal balance does not stabilize for several weeks, be aware of continuing joint laxity (looseness). It takes

about 12 weeks for joint and ligament laxity to return to normal after pregnancy.

5. Fatigue is a common problem for new mothers. If you are tired, it might be better to take a nap than to exercise. This is especially true if you are nursing.

6. Often, women are surprised to find they are incontinent after delivery. This can last for several months. The best exercises to correct this condition are Kegels (see page 212).

7. Sometimes the cumulative effects of pregnancy, labor, and carrying a baby lead to back pain. Watch your posture. Abdominal strengthening exercises may help (see precautions on page 205).

8. Take time to warm up and stretch before exercise, and give yourself an ample cool-down and relaxation period after exercise.

9. Nursing mothers should be particularly conscientious to drink lots of fluids. Finding a bra that provides breast support during exercise is also important.

10. Be sure to practice good nutritional habits. Though it may be inconvenient to eat properly when you have a small baby and a busy schedule, it's worth the effort. There is also no reason to rush weight loss, especially if you are nursing. Breast-feeding women lose weight more slowly because of the body's protective mechanisms.

11. Scheduling will take some juggling. Many women find it is difficult to make child care arrangements and/or to find the time to exercise in the early months; don't hesitate to ask your partner or a friend to help out. Your mental and physical health are important.

12. Relax and enjoy yourself! A brisk walk with your baby may be all you can do at first. As you develop a routine and can fit in regular exercise, you will find it provides important time for yourself.

TAKING AN ACTIVE ROLE IN YOUR PREGNANCY

Attitudes toward women and their bodies are changing. Pregnancy is no longer viewed as a disease state or a time when women are expected to be incapacitated. Few women "take to their beds" when they become pregnant; instead, many are simply buying a larger pair of workout clothes and continuing to exercise.

Pat Kulpa's research confirms that cardiovascular fitness can actually be improved by exercising while you're pregnant. Even so, many of the specific questions relating to physiology and the effects of exercise during pregnancy have yet to be resolved. If you're pregnant today, you may feel as if you can't wait until science has "all the answers."

The decisions you make about your lifestyle during pregnancy are personal ones. Because of our society's emphasis on fitness, you may feel as much pressure to exercise during pregnancy as not to exercise. As a pregnant woman, you naturally feel a responsibility to your growing child. You also need support for your decisions and actions. At Melpomene, we encourage women to take an active role in managing their pregnancies. We know, however, that not everything can be controlled. The experience of pregnancy, as well as labor and delivery, cannot be predicted. No one can guarantee a perfect pregnancy, or a wished-for pregnancy outcome. No matter how carefully you try to make healthy choices, the unexpected can happen. Remember that exercise is only one of many variables, known and unknown, that can influence the course of a pregnancy.

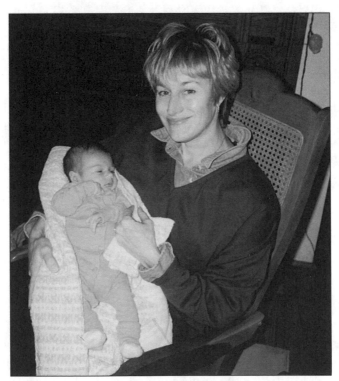

Gayle Winegar—whom we met on page 196—shown here with the end result of her healthy pregnancy.

Over and over again, women have told us that exercise helped make their pregnancies enjoyable. Many women have also said that the questions they asked and adjustments they made in their physical activity during pregnancy helped them remember how to enjoy exercise. They stressed that it made them feel good psychologically and physically. During pregnancy, exercise also helps maintain a good body image because it gives women a sense of control over their bodies at a time when many uncontrollable physical changes are occurring.

Pregnancy is also a time to think about priorities. We hope that the steps you take to ensure a healthy pregnancy are steps that will lead you to a healthy lifestyle long after your baby is born.

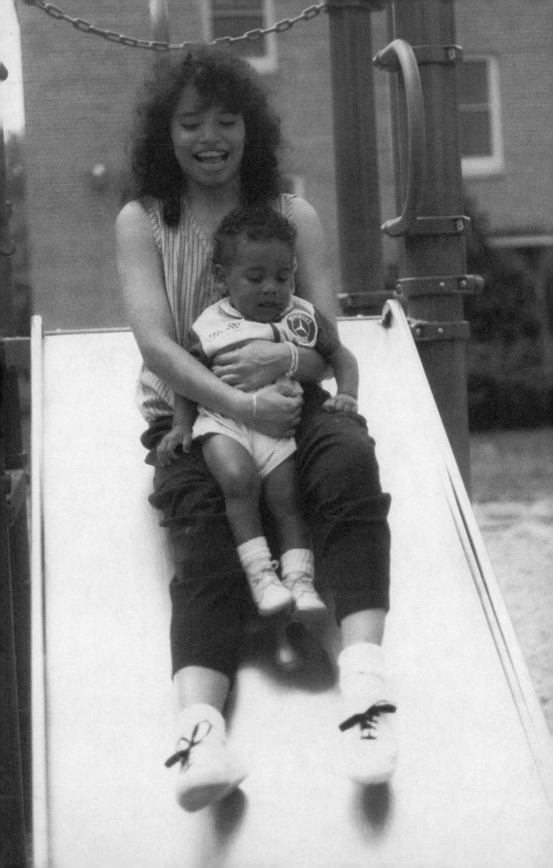

6

Your Child's Fitness

Monica's son, Derek, has just turned 3. Although Monica works most of the day and is tired when she gets home at 5:30, she tries to do something with Derek every evening. Sometimes she takes him to the park to play, but other times she stays closer to home and finds less active ways to keep Derek busy. Monica's worried that Derek might not be getting enough exercise. She wants to help him build good habits. She wonders, how much exercise should a child be getting?

Kendra's 7-year-old daughter, Tori, has been asking to play soccer on a local girls' team. Kendra signed Tori up on a team sponsored by the recreation center but still wonders if Tori is ready for organized sports. Kendra sees how competitive the sport can get and how some of the children tease the kids who seem a little slower than others. Is this the kind of activity Kendra wants her daughter involved with?

Our doctors, health officials, and even entertainers have become evangelical in recent years about the benefits of a physically active lifestyle. By now, most adults are aware of the many good reasons they should tear themselves away from TV and start to exercise: weight control, improved appearance, greater capacity and endurance for work and recreation, reduced stress, socializing opportunities, and generally enhanced well-being. But how many adults think about the benefits their children might gain through regular exercise, recreation, and sport? How many parents consider it their responsibility to encourage and facilitate physical activity for their kids?

But aren't children active enough? Many of us have vivid memories of an active childhood—long days of running, biking, swimming, and playing kickball in the school yard. We assume that children today must also get enough exercise in their normal patterns of play. Some kids do in fact stay fit by playing and participating in family recreation or organized sports; however, recent studies show that too many children are spending their days in front of the TV or video monitor, or in equally passive activities.

A growing number of health fitness professionals, teachers, coaches, and parents are concerned about this sedentary "couch potato" lifestyle. Too many children and adolescents are steering away from active pursuits such as swimming, hiking, bicycling, sports teams, skiing, and the myriad other physical activities available.

Are today's kids really less fit than the children of 20 years ago? Steven Blair, Director of Epidemiology at the Cooper Institute for Aerobics Research in Dallas, estimates that nationally 20 percent of children are at risk for premature death as adults due to low levels of fitness. However, physical activity experts also tell us that it is difficult to measure physical fitness in today's children because the definition of fitness has changed dramatically during the past decade. Today physical activity experts are concerned with a broader, long-term definition of fitness or "health-related physical fitness." The framework of health-related fitness is the reduction of cardiovascular risk factors and development of physical activity as a lifelong habit.

During the sixties and seventies fitness testing consisted of measures such as the long jump, softball throw, and 40-yard dash. These were mostly measures of power, speed, and agility—or motor ability. Today, however, we're more likely to assess fitness differently in our children, by measuring cardiorespiratory endurance, body composition, flexibility, and muscular endurance, most of which do not compare to the measures of 20 years ago.

What we *do* know is that the children of today are getting fatter. Several researchers are finding that children weigh more and have more body fat than did children 20 to 30 years ago. A study published in 1995 conducted by the National Center for Health Statistics of nearly 3,000 children nationally concluded that 11 percent of children aged 6 through 17 are severely overweight, more than twice the rate in the 1960s.

Most physical activity experts would also agree that kids are spending too much time with TV and video games. A 1992 survey sponsored by the International Food Information Council reported that on Saturdays and after school, 53 percent of the children in the study said they played outside, but 80 percent also said they watched TV. Not only does time in front of the TV interfere with time for physical activity, but TV watching may also contribute to obesity in children. Resting metabolic rate has been found to drop significantly during as little as 25 minutes of television viewing, and to make matters worse, children are bombarded with TV advertising encouraging consumption of high-calorie, high-fat snacks.

This situation requires action on the part of parents, coaches, and educators. Regardless of how fit or unfit our children are, it's not enough for us to rely on children's so-called natural inclination toward physical activity for lifetime fitness. Simply being "a kid" does not automatically make your child physically fit, nor will it prevent or reduce the risk that he or she will develop heart disease as an adult. Regular physical activity can help minimize these risk factors and can also set up a healthy habit that will carry over into adulthood.

How, then, do you as a parent help your child get involved in and excited about physical activity? What if you and your spouse or partner have not yet made exercise a regular part of your life: How do you figure out what will motivate your child?

As a parent, you are in a unique position of knowing your child better than anyone else and how best to help him or her understand the joys of physical activity. This chapter covers the benefits of being active for kids. It offers suggestions on how you, as a parent, can help your child develop physical activity as a lifelong habit, evaluate competitive sports for your child, and avoid participation dropout in your adolescent.

THE BENEFITS OF PHYSICAL ACTIVITY FOR CHILDREN

As with adults, regular physical activity provides a multitude of physical, psychological, and social benefits for kids. William Strong, MD, pediatrics professor and director of the Georgia Institute for the Prevention of Human Disease and Accidents, and Jack Wilmore, PhD, kinesiology professor at the University of Texas at Austin, have written about the many ways they believe children can benefit from regular physical activity and, ultimately, from physical fitness.

They tell us that regular activity can:

- control weight;
- control mild hypertension;

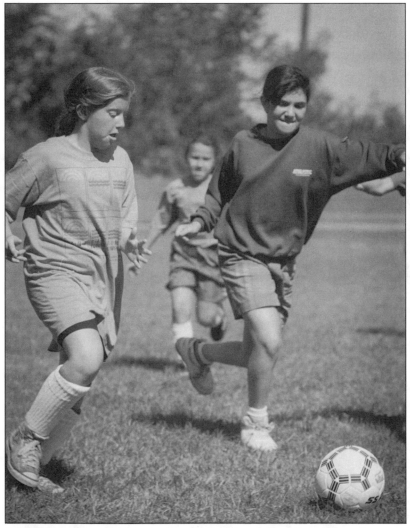

When they succeed physically, children grow in self-worth and appreciation of their bodies.

- improve posture;
- improve appearance;
- improve overall functional and motor abilities; and
- create a greater sense of psychological well-being and lower anxiety levels.

These and many other benefits of physical activity for children were confirmed by Melpomene's research. Findings indicate that children—from toddlers to teenagers—who are physically active are more likely to have better overall physical health, coordination, motor development, strength, flexibility, and regular sleeping patterns. Active kids also tend to recuperate more quickly from illness. Likewise, children who are active at a moderate level develop aerobic capacity for healthier heart and lungs, especially during adolescence.

The psychological benefits of participating in sports and recreational activities are also important. Mastering an activity can give kids self-confidence while enhancing their body image as well as their self-esteem. Their sense of accomplishment grows each time they take on and succeed in a new physical challenge. As they watch themselves improve, children begin to appreciate their bodies and trust their own physical potential. Once children get a sense of how good it feels to be fit, they will have a built-in incentive to keep exercising, even into adulthood.

The social benefits of participating in physical activities are also numerous. Through informal, active games or organized sports, children learn to get along with others, work as part of a team, and handle losing or failure. When the entire family participates, the relationships between parents and children are usually enhanced. These social skills will serve children later in life, when they may function more effectively as part of an office team or when they are developing relationships with their own children.

WHAT INFLUENCES CHILDREN'S PHYSICAL ACTIVITY PATTERNS?

Leah's 5-year-old, Hannah, is constantly on the go. She rides her bike around the neighborhood every day and asks to go swimming every weekend. Hannah can't wait to be a year older so she can join a youth softball team.

Despite his parents' efforts, Daryl, at age 9, would prefer to watch
TV most of the time. His mom enrolled Daryl in a swim program,
but after the program was over, Daryl was not interested in continuing. Daryl also tried karate for a while but, again, did not like
the classes enough to keep it up.

Why is there such a disparity in activity levels for these children?
What contributes to making some girls and boys so much more active
than their counterparts? It appears that the combined influences of
family, community, and school contribute significantly to whether and
how extensively children become and remain physically active.

Parents

Brothers Mark, age 6, and Terry, age 10, like to ride bikes. However, they don't ride for very long around their neighborhood.
After about 10 minutes of riding, both Mark's and Terry's bikes end
up back in the garage, and the boys are looking for some other
game to play. Occasionally, their mom will take Mark and Terry for
a ride on a nearby bike trail, where both boys will ride for several
miles, racing each other and enjoying the scenery. Usually when
it is time to turn around and start for home, the boys will ask to ride
even farther.

A primary reason children are active is simply to have fun. This was
one conclusion of a 1993 study conducted by Renee Stucky-Ropp and
Thomas DiLorenzo at the University of Missouri. In their study to
determine what influences children to be physically active, the researchers talked with 242 fifth- and sixth-grade children and their
mothers about their attitudes toward sports and physical activity. They
found that the best predictors for kids to be active in sports was
enjoyment, as well as the mother's attitudes and friends' and family's
support for physical activity. Parents' own physical activity and the
number of sports or exercise-related items found at home were also
important contributors to a child's level of activity.

Parents can exert a very positive influence on their children's physical activity and fitness levels in a variety of ways. Encouragement from
parents is a strong motivator for children to participate in an activity,
and physical activity is no exception. A few positive words about a
newly learned skill or about how hard your child worked at a physical

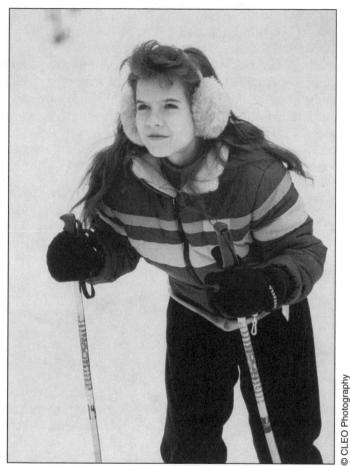

© CLEO Photography

What's the main reason that kids are active? Because it's fun.

task may be motivation enough for the child to want to continue or repeat that activity.

More powerful, however, than verbal support, is a parent's role modeling of a physically active lifestyle. Several studies have documented that more physically active parents have more active children, from preschoolers to adolescents.

A survey conducted at Melpomene also found that children who had more physically active mothers also had higher physical activity levels. We asked all mothers in this study to rate how much of an impact, if any, various factors had on their child's participation in physical activities and sports. The most highly ranked positive influences were mothers' and fathers' own physical activity patterns. Children who see their parents jog in the neighborhood or ride their bikes for transportation and recreation, or hear about how much they enjoy their tennis matches or cross-country ski trips, tend to get a positive image of physical activity.

Equally as important as physically active parents are parents who make movement a priority as a family. Time spent engaged in family activities as simple as walking, biking, or playing kickball are powerful examples and deliver the message that an active lifestyle is important for everyone.

You can also influence your child's physical activity through environmental factors in the following ways:

- Encouraging them to play outdoors. Children's movement tends to be limited indoors. If you send your child outdoors, he or she is likely to find an active game to play.
- Limiting your child's television viewing. Again, if they are not sitting in front of the TV, they will likely find something more active to do.
- Having the right kinds of toys. A good supply of balls of all sizes, a jump rope, a sled, roller skates, or ice skates can make outdoor play more appealing.
- Having access to facilities. This can be as simple as a neighborhood skating rink, an open field for kite flying or kickball, or some gym time at a local school.

How Can Parents Encourage Children's Physical Activity?

As parents we can be powerful motivators for our children's activity patterns. But what exactly can we do to encourage our children to be physically active? By setting good examples and providing encouragement and opportunities, we can open the door to children across all age ranges for enjoyable, safe, and health-enhancing recreation and sports.

Here are some positive actions you can take:

Through Family Activities

- Set an example; be active yourself.
- Make time for physical activity and recreation as a family.
- Invite children to walk or bike with you as an alternative to travel by car.

(cont.)

How Can Parents Encourage Children's Physical Activity?
(cont.)

- Include children on camping, hiking, canoeing, skiing, and other trips and outings.
- Promote lifelong sports such as swimming, cycling, tennis, jogging, skiing, or hiking.

Through Support

- Show enthusiasm and support for children's accomplishments without expecting superior athletic achievements.
- Help your children set goals that are reasonable and achievable for their age, physical maturation, psychological readiness, and individual physical abilities.
- Encourage activities that do not involve excessive competition, training, or physical contact beyond their physical or psychological capabilities.
- Find the right sport for your child. This may involve trying a variety of activities to find the one or two that best suit your child.

Through Discussion

- Talk to your children about their specific interests, and let them choose activities they enjoy most.
- Discuss and provide opportunities for taking lessons or classes, going to camp, or joining scouting clubs offering physical activities.
- Talk to children about how they are feeling—physically and emotionally—to help avoid potential injuries or emotional anxieties stemming from sports participation.
- Emphasize enjoyment and personal improvement over "win, win, win" or "no pain, no gain."

Community Opportunities and Children's Interests

Factors outside the home can also have significant positive influences on children's involvement in physical activity. Among them are community recreation programs, sports lessons and classes, extracurricular school sports programs, and access to recreational facilities such as parks, softball fields, skating rinks, and swimming pools. Parents play a valuable role here, too, by finding out what programs and facilities are available, discussing their children's interests, encouraging them to participate, and taking an ongoing interest in their experiences with these activities.

Other variables also have important, positive influences on children's sports and recreation patterns. As might be expected, children with good overall health and good athletic skills are more inclined to be physically active. However, many parents who responded to our survey said their children had substantial interest in physical activities despite their small size, lagging muscle development, or lack of physical

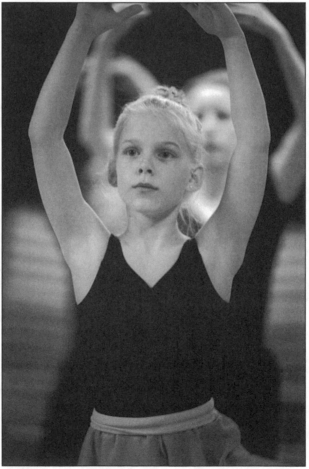

© Terry Wild Studio

Look in your community for programs to keep your child busy, happy, and challenged.

abilities. If a child has a risk-taking or assertive personality, or if his or her parents strongly reinforce each achievement, the child can often overcome disadvantages in physical stature, skill, or ability.

Gender

Regardless of size or ability, the sex of your child may also have an impact on his or her level of physical activity. Gender can influence participation in physical activity in many ways. At an early age, children learn what are appropriate games, toys, and activities for their gender. Boys' toys are typically action-oriented. Toys such as action figures illustrate the strength and power of the male superhero. Toys for girls typically emphasize appearance. Children get the message that boys should be powerful and active, and girls should be physically attractive rather than physically active.

This stereotype carries over into sports, where traditionally men have been the sports heroes while women cheer from the sidelines. While this is changing, historically sport has been defined as appropriate for males and inappropriate for females. A 1995 report released by the Feminist Majority Foundation highlights the fact that while the situation is in flux, women in athletics still have a long way to go toward equality with men. They report that women receive only 30 percent of college athletic scholarship money, and that women are allowed to participate in only 86 summer Olympic events, compared with men's 159.

Tiffany, age 13, describes how her parents think sports are more important for her brother than for her.

> "My brother can do whatever he wants in sports, but I have to be school smart and get good grades. My parents have given my brother chances that I never would have gotten. He plays baseball and basketball really well. My brother gets to do all of those things, and my mom tells me I never started so why start now?"

We can move toward changing this inequality and stereotyping through our own modeling and teaching children, both girls *and* boys, about gender differences. By modeling flexibility in our actions and ideas, we can eliminate the idea that some activities are gender-incongruous. Parents and other adults can teach children that activities and objects are not gender-specific, allowing children to develop in areas that may otherwise be restricted because of their gender.

Getting your children involved in sports and recreation is a great way to help them cultivate a lifelong physical habit. The benefits are far-reaching in terms of immediate and long-term gains in health and well-being. Help them discover that fitness is fun!

PHYSICAL EDUCATION

The cost and availability of out-of-school sports programs may limit some children's participation. For many children physical education in school may be their only opportunity to engage in regular physical activity. Therefore physical education programs promoting cardiovascular health and lifelong fitness are imperative.

Unfortunately, not all kids take physical education in school, especially as they advance to the middle and high school grades. A national survey of 16,296 high school students nationally, conducted by the U.S. Department of Health and Human Services, concluded that only 52 percent of youths in grades 9 through 12 are enrolled in physical education classes; only 34 percent of the students had physical education classes daily.

Even for those children who do have physical education classes as part of their school curriculum, we must ask, is the allotted time given to those classes enough to develop fitness? Given the average class period of about 30 to 40 minutes, and allowing time for class management and instruction, fitness experts estimate that only 5 to 15 minutes of class time is spent engaged in moderate to vigorous physical activity.

Additionally, parents, physical educators, and fitness experts are divided as to the primary objective of PE classes. Should classes focus on developing fitness to the exclusion of skill development? Or should skill development be taught, with less time given to aerobic activities? Increasing skills without an emphasis on fitness is not likely to lead to lifelong physical activity. The best solution is a combination of moderate to vigorous aerobic activities that incorporate skill development.

Childhood fitness experts offer several ways for physical educators to accomplish this goal. Classes that integrate drills with game play, organize games with small numbers of students to increase participation times, or devote a portion of each class specifically to the development of cardiovascular fitness achieve this objective.

Researchers are finding that programs focusing on fitness are in fact producing fitter kids. Several studies have concluded that physical education curriculums devoted to aerobic activity produced improvement in cardiovascular fitness, physical activity levels inside and outside of school, and reduced cardiovascular risk factors in those children participating.

So, how does an educator make gym time fun? Parents may be concerned that physical education classes focusing on aerobic activity may turn their children off to physical activity. Grant Hill, an assistant professor in the School of Physical Education and Athletics at Seattle Pacific University, devised the PASS Approach for Games and Relays for children in kindergarten through grade six. The PASS Approach stands for Protection, Alternatives, Stimulation, and Sensitivity, and ensures that children play in a safe, appropriate way, while emphasizing fitness. Hill suggests:

- Protection: This involves playing in a safe environment, giving kids space to play, staying away from walls, avoiding rough games, and full supervision.
- Alternatives: Educators may need to modify games to develop certain skills, to alter the level of challenge, or even to include other subjects such as math or science.
- Stimulation: In order to optimize aerobic activity in the allotted time, kids need to keep moving. Games should involve smaller teams for increased participation; avoid elimination games, and try to keep waiting time to a minimum.
- Sensitivity: In order for children of varying skills to participate, educators need to de-emphasize winning and losing, avoid picking teams, put slower students in the middle of relay teams, and switch team members often.

While it's a tall order to fill, physical educators who can be flexible and attentive to the abilities of all students while focusing on total fitness provide an environment in which all students have an opportunity to be successful. Such a positive physical education experience lays a foundation for fit children to grow into fit adults.

ORGANIZED SPORTS AND COMPETITION

Once your child has developed fundamental skills and shows an interest, you and your child may decide to give organized sports a try. Organized sports teams are sponsored by a variety of institutions or agencies, including schools, youth organizations, and clubs. They usually involve a series of practices and games at a variety of skill levels. Teams vary by cost, competitive level, length of season, and focus of coaching staff. Team sports are a great way for youngsters to develop their skills and gain confidence. Participating in team sports can also teach a child about sportsmanship, teamwork, and friendship.

Research conducted by Vern Seefeldt and his colleagues at the Youth Sports Institute at Michigan State University finds that both boys and girls participate in school and nonschool sports primarily to have fun. In nonschool sports, boys say participation for fun is followed by the ability to do something at which they're good and to improve their skills. After fun, girls say they participate to stay in shape and to get exercise.

A common misconception is that kids participate in sports primarily to compete. The results of Seefeldt's study help to disprove this belief. Girls in this study ranked the challenge of competition tenth on their list of reasons for participating, and boys ranked competition sixth. A 1991 Melpomene focus group study of adolescent girls confirmed that competition is not a strong motivator for girls to be physically active. In fact, some girls talked about being intimidated by competition and avoided those situations altogether.

Parents, coaches, and other adults who work with youngsters disagree somewhat as to how much competition is healthy. In general, parents need to take into account their child's personality and age in determining if that child is emotionally and physically ready for serious competition. Too much too soon can sour a child's attitude toward organized sports, causing the child to avoid them in the future. Bear in mind that the benefits of organized sports are to build physical skills, learn about teamwork and good sportsmanship, have fun, and establish physical activity as a habit. It's true that some of these skills are learned through winning and losing, but an intense focus on winning will overwhelm most children.

Both parents and coaches play a critical role in the lifelong attitudes that children develop toward sports. Most parents and coaches take a healthy interest in their child's sports activities. However, sometimes adults tend to push children into sports situations before they are ready. Occasionally, adult forms of "encouragement" become too vehement, and children may believe that their personal worth hinges on winning and sport performance.

One talented athlete, Nicole, loved the sport of volleyball and looked forward to each practice and game. Nicole's mother, however, had a different attitude toward her daughter's participation. To Nicole's mother, the sport was a serious undertaking, and winning each game was the only acceptable outcome. Not only that, but Nicole's mother pushed her to be the star of the team. Ultimately, because of her mother's attitude, Nicole lost the joy of playing volleyball. At the end of the season, she questioned if she would ever play again.

Why Kids Drop Out of Sports

The reasons why children drop out of youth sports programs are varied. Researchers in this area have arrived at different conclusions, depending on the subject's age, gender, sport, and type of program.

It is important for parents to remember that sport dropout is not necessarily negative, nor is it necessarily permanent. For many children what is perceived as a drop from one sport is merely a transfer to a different sport at a later time. Dropout from sports programs is normal and occurs regularly, especially as children move through the adolescent and high school years.

Among the reasons:
- Conflicts arise with other interests, such as other clubs or work.
- Your child is no longer interested in the sport.
- Your child is not having fun.
- Too much pressure is associated with the sport.
- Your child needs more time to study.
- Your child has a conflict with a coach (not enough play time, coach plays favorites, coach is a poor teacher).
- Too much emphasis is placed on winning.
- Your child is tired of playing.

As a parent, it is important that you keep the channels of communication open with your child. Regardless of the reason for wanting to drop out, your child will likely have some concerns, and will be looking to you to support his or her decision.

From Seefeldt 1992, Weiss 1989.

As a parent or coach, you can help ensure your children's enjoyment and continued participation by keeping the following guidelines in mind.

- Emphasize skill development by helping your child choose performance goals that are realistic. This allows the young athlete to control the consequences of his or her actions and focus on improvement. For example, you may encourage your daughter to improve her follow-through on basketball shots, increasing her chances for scoring, rather than focusing on the scoring itself. Stress both individual and team priorities.

- Teach your child that winning isn't everything in sports. While winning is important, most kids would rather play regularly on a losing team than sit on the bench of a winning team. Taking pride in having done their best is more valuable to children in the long run than winning.
- Be sure that the team for which you are signing your child up is a good match for your child. What is the skill level of the players? What are the goals the coaching staff has for the team? If there is not a good fit between your child and the team, he or she may come away from the experience feeling discouraged, rather than eager to sign up again next season.
- Praise your child's efforts. Children who receive positive comments develop positive self-esteem and enjoy sports more than those who do not.
- Keep organized sports fun. Children participate in sports because it is fun. Having a good time can be the determinant of whether your child will continue to participate or not.
- Listen to what your child is telling you about the sport experience and how well it is working. Take action or make changes as appropriate.

Tips on Getting Along With Your Child's Coach

Eva Sipkins, mother of two boys who are active in organized hockey, baseball, tennis, and soccer, offers the following suggestions for dealing with your child's coach.

- Remember that coaches are often parents, usually working in a volunteer capacity. Their experience may be limited, and coaching may be a learning process for them as well as for their athletes.
- Don't judge a coach by one game. Try to get to as many games and practices as you can.
- Parents should understand that at each age level, kids are taught specific skills. The focus is guided by the governing association for each sport. Be aware of what the task is for your child for that particular season.

(cont.)

Tips on Getting Along With Your Child's Coach (cont.)

- Different levels of a sport may have different rules. Parents are usually given a set of the rules at the beginning of each season. If you do not receive one, ask for a copy. Be sure to read them.
- If you see the coach doing something you don't like, don't jump in immediately. Wait and see; the coach may catch himself or herself and make the change independently. If you do say something, suggest—don't ever yell.
- If the coach on an opposing team exhibits poor sportsmanship, a good plan of action is to have several parents call the governing association.
- Don't criticize your child's coach in front of your child. This undermines the coach's authority in your child's eyes.
- If you are having a hard time talking to the coach or feel that you are not being heard, you might try to establish a relationship with the assistant coach. A head coach might be more likely to listen to an assistant coach than to a parent.
- Be sure to model good sportsmanship if you expect your child to be a good sport. After one angry outburst, Eva's son reminded her, "Mom, remember those rules— they're for parents, too."
- Let the coach know you appreciate his or her efforts. If your child is learning and having fun, the coach is doing a good job.

Too Much, Too Soon? Minimizing Negative Experiences

So far, it would appear that the benefits of physical activity far outweigh any disadvantages or negative impacts. However, a focus on activities that are overly competitive or developmentally too complicated for young children only serves to frustrate children and turn them away from participation. By keeping in mind a few basic considerations,

Renell Pettinelli: Coaching Is Rewarding

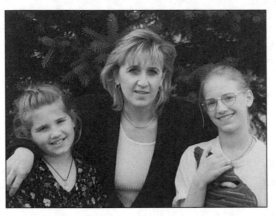

Becoming a coach wasn't an easy decision for me," says Renell Pettinelli. "It meant giving up an aerobics class I had just started. I was finally doing something for myself. But my daughters wanted to play pitchball, and they couldn't find anyone else to coach."

Renell's mom never coached her. "My family was not sports-minded, but I joined the volleyball team in high school and became a good player. I wanted my daughters to be able to start sports much earlier.

"When I coach, I stress fun, building self-esteem, and developing skills. But beginning players can be rough on a coach who wants to build self-esteem. Once my team lost by 50 runs. Around the third inning, I really just wanted to go home. You know the kids have potential, and you know what abilities are there, but the abilities didn't come through.

"Fortunately, winning isn't the only way to improve self-esteem. One day I went home and made a list of all the players and wrote something positive about what each one had done during the game. I read the list the next time the team got together. As I read aloud what each player had done, the kids cheered for each other. I thought that was great. If you can't feel good about yourself, if you don't start with that, then you just aren't going to get anywhere.

"Another thing that keeps me coming back to coaching is to see some of my players develop skills and self-confidence. I had one player who struggled to keep up with the others when they ran around the field. There would be this big group of girls, then a big space, then Erin. But, by the end of the season, she was running right along with them. I love to see that kind of progress."

Is Renell glad she's a coaching mom? "You bet." Does she regret giving up her aerobics class? "Not at all. It has been amazing for me to see how important coaches are in the lives of these girls. Coaching goes way beyond just teaching skills. It includes teaching good manners and caring for each other. And they listen to everything you say. I hope that the girls on my team will continue playing sports for the rest of their lives."

parents, physicians, teachers, and coaches can minimize or avoid negative consequences and can help make sports and recreation positive experiences for children.

It is important for parents to remember that children have shorter attention spans than teenagers or adults, and this needs to be considered when choosing a sport for your child. Sports or activities that require a great deal of concentration, such as golf or baseball, may not be the best choice for younger children. Also, sports that demand long periods of time for practice may also leave youngsters feeling bored and frustrated.

Each child develops at his or her own pace, and this also applies as children acquire sports skills. Not only does physical readiness need to be considered, but psychological and social development must be taken into account as well. Burt, the father of an 8-year-old son, Andy, found this to be true after enrolling Andy in a summer soccer program. After the first couple of practices, Burt noticed his son falling behind in most of the drills. As a result, Andy was becoming frustrated and losing confidence. In talking with the coaches, Burt realized that Andy was not developmentally ready to play with this age group. He was too young to understand some of the drill concepts, as well as being socially and emotionally immature for the disciplined interactions needed to play soccer at that level.

Clearly, not every sport is appropriate for a 5-year-old. Likewise, a 14-year-old will be easily disinterested with an activity that is too simple and lacks challenge. Finding activities that match your child's level of development and maturity will increase the likelihood of an enjoyable sport experience and will encourage him or her to stay involved for a lifetime. The following list describes sports skills at various levels of childhood development.

With a little imagination, you can modify activities to fit your child's abilities. For example, using balloons instead of balls may make a game of catch more fun for your 3-year-old. Other modifications for young children might include making larger goals or targets. For example, use a waste basket or large wall targets. Using soft balls such as a Nerf or yarn ball reduces a child's fear of getting hurt while learning to catch. Also consider that games that require running or hopping could be played while walking. For older children, modifications for more developmentally appropriate play might include a smaller playing field, modified scoring, or altered team size.

As children grow older, they acquire more sophisticated skills, but it is important for parents to remember that even through adolescence, children are continuing to develop motor skills. Beyond age appropriateness, however, parents of adolescents are faced with new challenges and

Sports Skills and Childhood Development

Infancy (0 to 2 years): Basic motor reflex skills are being developed during this time. Basic skills such as walking and climbing are also developed. Free play is recommended for exploration and movement within a safe environment.

Early Childhood (2 to 5 years): These children are beginning to develop basic motor skills, such as kicking, throwing, running, and hopping. Playfulness and exploration are important at this age. Simple, fun activities such as running, tumbling, tossing, and catching are recommended.

Childhood (5 to 9 years): Basic motor skills are continuing to develop. Some organized activities may be appropriate, depending on the child's level of readiness. Competition should not be emphasized during this time. Running, swimming, and gymnastics are good choices. Some older children may be ready for the high skill level and quick decision-making necessary for sports such as hockey, basketball, and football.

Late Childhood (9 to 12 years): Separate skills, once developed, can be used in conjunction with other skills for children in this age group. For example, a running kick utilizes both running form and kicking skill. Most entry-level activities are appropriate for these children. Organized sports practices should be kept short, and competition and overtraining should be avoided.

Source: Nelson, 1991; Kolata, 1992; and Bunker, 1991.

pleasures as their children move to more advanced levels of physical activity.

CHILDREN WITH DISABILITIES

Parents of children with disabilities often wonder how they can best encourage their child to be physically active. Martin E. Block, PhD, at the Curry School of Education, University of Virginia, makes the following recommendations:

- Listen to your child's interest. Allow your child to choose not to play a particular sport. Some children gravitate toward sports with which they feel more comfortable or that they want to try.
- Be encouraging and supportive. Children, even children without disabilities, will make mistakes. Let your children know that it is OK to make mistakes and that you will still love them regardless of their performance. In fact, let them know that the best way to learn and improve is by making mistakes.
- Encourage your child to practice on his or her own. Determine what equipment and setup your child needs to practice independently, and then help with this arrangement. Reinforce your child whenever he or she chooses to practice an activity independently.
- Help your child set realistic goals and expectations. Not everyone can be a star of the team. Your child's goals should be realistic and achievable. On the other hand, do not squelch your child's enthusiasm and dreams.
- Talk about athletes with disabilities who can serve as role models (e.g., Jim Abbott, pitcher for the California Angels who has one arm; Jackie Joyner-Kersee, Olympic heptathlon champion who has severe asthma). You can also help your child identify role models closer to home who are more accessible.
- Don't push your child; be sure he or she is mentally and physically prepared. This does not mean waiting for your child to achieve a level of skillfulness and understanding that he or she may never achieve. Rather, choose leagues and activities that match your child's abilities. In more advanced programs, provide support to your child such as assisting during practice and in games.
- Encourage your child to try different sports. Before allowing your child to say "no" to certain sports, help him or her make an informed decision. For example, rent a video or take the child to see the sport being played before allowing a refusal. Promote activity in both team and individual sports—try not to favor one over the other.
- Use equipment that is appropriate for your child's age, physical characteristics, and abilities. For example:
  —Use bigger, softer balls for beginners who are learning to catch and kick.

—Set up stationary targets for striking and throwing.
—Use smaller balls for small hands when throwing.
—Use smaller racquets or other striking implements when striking.
—Slow down the speed of the object being caught or hit (use balloons, scarves, or beach balls).
—Establish smaller playing areas for low endurance.
—Lower goals (basketball).
—Make goals bigger (soccer).
—Provide for lots of turns (use small teams and more than one ball).

• Be an advocate within the public school system for appropriate physical education programs for all children. Evaluate your child's PE program—ask to see a sample of the curriculum in elementary and secondary PE. Discuss any specific gross motor goals that your child's PE teacher has for the children over the course of the year.

HELPING YOUR DAUGHTER BECOME ACTIVE

You might find it more difficult to interest your adolescent daughter than your adolescent son. Often girls do not receive encouragement to be active or hear the message that sports are as important to girls as they are to boys. Moreover, girls often face fewer opportunities to play on sports teams than boys. For that reason, the rest of this chapter focuses on issues related to girls and sport.

The Adolescent Years

The teenage years can be an emotional roller coaster. As girls move from childhood to adulthood, it can feel as if the whole world is watching, and that girls' very worth depends on whether or not they are popular. Peer groups become the critical panel of experts, setting the bounds for what is acceptable and, more important, what is "cool."

In addition, the adolescent years can be a time when self-confidence seems to disappear. A 1990 study conducted by the American Association of University Women found that as girls move through adolescence, their self-esteem drops sharply, a drop far more pronounced for girls than for boys. Harvard researcher Carol Gilligan and her

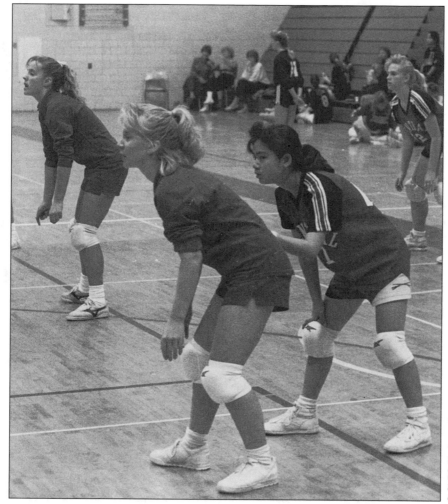

© CLEO Photography

Once adolescence hits, girls tend to decrease sport participation—and thus miss out on the corresponding positive self-esteem.

colleagues suggest reasons for this decline: Adolescent girls are more likely to make relationship-based decisions. As a result, girls tend to be more susceptible than boys to what others think, becoming concerned with being good and being liked.

The adolescent years are also a time of declining sports participation, especially for girls. At Melpomene, we see a link between these two findings. Having studied the reasons for and benefits of physical activity for women from 1982 to 1990, we are well aware of the relationship between physical activity and positive self-esteem. In light of this relationship and reports of declining adolescent self-esteem, in

1990 we were compelled to ask, "If teenage girls are dropping out of sports, are they missing out on the positive benefit of improved self-esteem associated with physical activity?"

In 1990-91 we began to study the relationship between sports participation and self-esteem in girls 9 to 17 years old. Data were collected through a questionnaire that determined self-esteem and physical activity levels. We also met in focus groups to collect data, so the girls could tell us firsthand about their feelings and experiences associated with physical activity.

Like women polled earlier, the girls in this study derived self-esteem from their participation in sports and physical activities. The girls who had the highest self-esteem scores were the ones who were physically active at the highest levels. They engaged in more sports and participated for longer time periods.

In the focus group setting, the girls talked a great deal about ways they gained self-esteem through sports. Many told about times they were challenged or took a risk. Others shared stories about achievement—not just winning, but learning a new skill or even being a member of a team. Still other girls shared their experiences of participating when friends or parents were watching, and of pride in other girls who were participating at a difficult level.

Despite the positive boost to self-esteem that many girls gained through sports, many of the girls in this study also talked about obstacles in the sports arena that often left them questioning their ability and self-worth. Most commonly, they described incidents involving boys who did not treat them as equal players. For example, they cited boys controlling the game, hogging the ball, picking the girls last for teams, or criticizing the girls if they made a mistake. Other girls spoke of other barriers to participation, including unequal treatment from PE teachers, lack of opportunity, lack of encouragement, and the lack of attention that girls' sports receive.

Is it any wonder that some girls are not as interested in sports as boys are? What can you as a parent or teacher do to encourage your teenage girls to be active? Possible strategies include:

- Provide opportunities for girls in all kinds of sports, including traditional male sports, such as football and hockey. Opportunities should be provided for players of all skill levels. Whenever possible, equipment should be supplied by the sponsoring agency to ensure that girls' participation will not be limited by finances.
- Encourage same-sex teams, on which girls can play and try new activities in an environment that is safe psychosocially

as well as physically. Choose a level of competition that is appropriate for the skill level and social development of a particular participant.

- Be aware of a girl's motivation for participating in a sport. Competition is not a primary reason for most girls. Girls are more likely to participate not only for fun, but also to socialize, build skills, and get in shape.
- Support girls' athletics by being a fan. Encouragement and approval are strong motivations for girls' sports participation.
- Encourage girls to speak out for increased opportunities for women and girls to engage in sports.
- Educate young boys about how and why they should support increasing girls' physical activity opportunities.

Co-Ed Versus Same-Sex Sports Teams

When your daughter decides she wants to participate in a sport, the decision must be made as to whether she should be on a co-ed or same-sex team. This decision can be based on her age, her reasons for participation, her skill level, and her interest in competition.

Prior to puberty, there are few physiological reasons for separate teams. After puberty, these differences become more of an issue. However, some would argue that boys usually have an advantage in skill level because many start earlier and receive more encouragement than girls. If teams are made up of boys and girls who are equal in skill, weight, and experience, then it is possible to have equitable co-ed teams.

Each type of team has its advantages. On a single-sex team, girls can learn the sport and develop their skills in a less critical environment. Leadership qualities may emerge more readily because girls feel less intimidated about taking the initiative in a group situation. Also, as a result of being on an all-girls team, girls play more often and spend less time sitting on the bench.

A co-ed team allows boys and girls to interact in a different way, and on the playing field, they must work together as well as compete against each other. Also, co-ed teams frequently allow for higher levels of competition.

Don't be afraid to ask the coach some questions. If the team is co-ed, it is important to find out how the team's members are chosen. For example, are there equal numbers of boys and girls on each team? Are team members selected according to their age, weight, or ability? Are the "best" kids picked first to be on the "A" teams, or are the teams

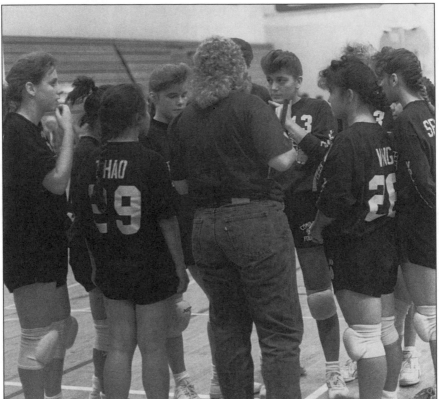

On a single-sex team, girls can learn the sport and develop their skills while feeling less pressured and less open to criticism.

divided randomly? Also, what are the goals or the focus of the team? Is the emphasis on winning, or for everyone to have fun and learn important skills?

Role Models

Exposing girls to female role models is an important component to developing lifelong physical activity habits. This ingredient is often missing. Role models are crucial because children see their heroes succeeding and picture themselves doing the same thing. Without role models, children often cannot envision themselves accomplishing their dreams, simply because they don't have anyone to inspire them.

Girls are frequently denied role models, especially in sports settings, a situation prevalent in all forms of the media. When she opens the sports pages of the local paper, your daughter is not likely to see much about local or national women's sports. She is also unlikely to hear much about women's sports when she turns on the TV, as women's sports receive only about 5 percent of late-night sports news coverage.

We don't even see enough physically active girls in children's literature either. In a 1993 Melpomene study looking at how girls are portrayed in children's books, girls were again underrepresented. Out of a random sample of 105 picture books with a sports theme, only 20 percent featured girls or women as dominant characters. However, 58 percent of the books contained males as the main characters. The message that girls are not good in sports or suited to sports was conveyed through the large number of stories in which males were the only characters or women were passive or peripheral figures.

Too often we assume that good role models for girls need to be well-known or Olympic athletes. This is not true. In a 1994 Melpomene study, we asked girls age 11 to 17 who they admire. We found that girls are far more likely to admire someone close to home, such as a parent or family member, than a famous athlete. This is not necessarily bad news. While girls may have fewer famous women athletes to admire, they have looked closer to home for role models. Yes, role models can be Olympic athletes, but they can also be mom or dad or the woman next door who loves to play hockey!

LIFELONG FITNESS

Throughout this chapter we've seen that children need encouragement to develop physical activity into a lifelong habit. While children's natural inclination is to be active, and physical education and organized sports are all steps toward this goal, the key is parental involvement and encouragement. As parents, you have the greatest impact in your child's fitness habits. By listening to and supporting your child and keeping sports safe and fun, you will have given your child the building blocks for a lifetime of activity.

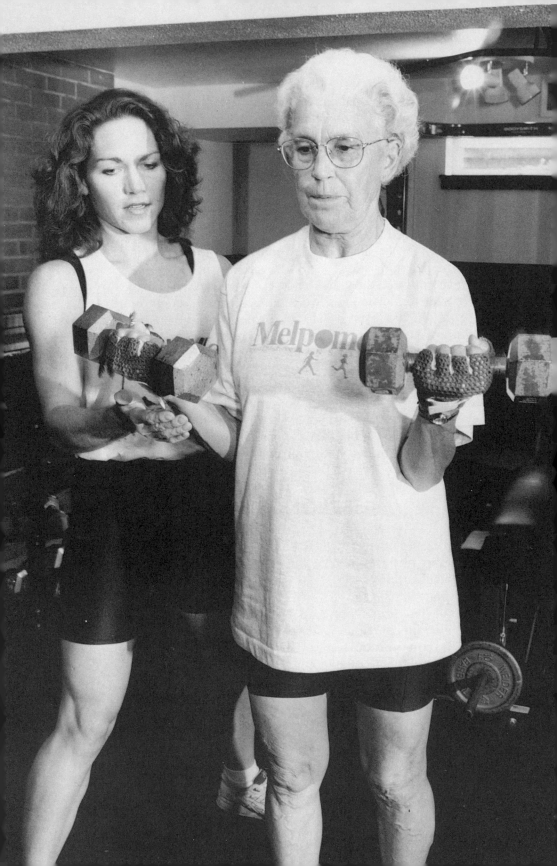

7

Age and the Active Woman

When she turned 68, Agnes retired from her job and told her son she needed a new hobby to keep busy and active. Her son suggested that she start a personalized workout program at a local fitness center. After a relatively sedentary life, Agnes felt recharged by the new activity. "I've never felt so alive," she says. "I should have started this 20 years ago!"

Paula has been active all her life. When she had major surgery at 65 to remove a tumor pressing against her spinal cord, one of her first questions after the surgery was, "When can I play tennis?" She says she knows she will feel much better, both physically and mentally, as soon as she can get active again. As she continues to recover from surgery, her longer daily walks are proof that she's progressing steadily.

WHAT CAN WE EXPECT?

When people say someone is "aging gracefully," they are usually referring to physical appearance. But the real secret of aging well has nothing to do with looks; it's all attitude. One of our members has a great comeback for women who are dreading the aging process. "If you're worried about getting old," she says, "just think of the alternative!"

Aging is part of moving forward in life, a process we all begin at birth. As women, we experience a second "coming of age" when there is a decrease in our hormones, signaling the end of our reproductive years and the beginning of menopause. This transition into a new stage of life is a time to consider our past struggles, our current abilities, and our future potential. In developed countries of the world, most women can expect to live 25 years or more after menopause. Women preparing for these years are inundated with articles and advertisements about special diets or exercise programs, many of which come with glowing "guarantees" for a healthier old age. Naturally, there is some confusion on the part of women who are trying to ferret out factual information about what they can do to enhance their later years.

You may have asked yourself some of these same questions: Will I have to slow down? Should I take calcium supplements? What about vitamin D? . . . protein? Can I start biking, swimming or skating at 60? How will physical activity affect my health? . . . my attitude? . . . my self-esteem? Will being active mean I'll look 10 years younger? In this chapter, we'll explore some of these questions by looking at the changes you can expect with aging and the role that becoming or staying active can play, as well as ways to alleviate menopausal discomfort and lessen your risk of osteoporosis and heart disease.

Lifestyle Changes

As our life span grows longer, the concept of aging takes on new meaning. Because life expectancies now stretch into the seventies and eighties, the "midlife" years creep into the fifties, and the sixties seem younger than they once did. At Melpomene, where we are privileged to work with very active senior volunteers and master athletes, we've learned to gauge a woman not by the number of years that she's been alive, but by how alive she feels, acts, and looks today.

In addition to the physical changes, which we'll discuss next, we can all look forward to some type of lifestyle change in our later years. After several decades of working and/or raising a family, a whole new segment of life can open up when the last child leaves or when retirement begins. If we have our health, there is no end to the new frontiers we can begin to explore. It can be a time for travel, for going back to school, or for realizing the dreams of a second career. It can also be a release from time pressures, when many women, perhaps for the first time, finally have time for themselves. For those of us who haven't ever made time for physical activity, the second half of life offers an excellent opportunity to start playing. There are many ways to combine travel and activity, such as walking tours, biking vacations, or other excursions. Grandchildren can be another wonderful entree to the world of play. They are built-in partners, and romping with them in the park or backyard can put us back in touch with our physical self.

Physical activity can also come in handy as a stress reducer in later years, when some of the changes we must face can feel beyond our control. Considering that most of us are likely to experience the death of a partner or close friend, a serious illness in our family or circle of friends, or divorce or separation in our later years, physical activity can be added to anyone's list of healthy ways to handle difficult times. In

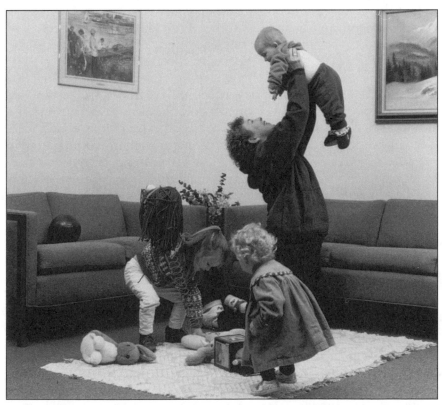

Grandchildren are built-in activity partners and playmates—take advantage!

fact, in a 1993 Melpomene/*Self* study of active women 40 to 60 years old, reported by Judy Mahle Lutter and Kathy Grumstrup in "Physical Activity and Weight in the Menopausal Years," physical activity was the most common method mentioned of reducing stress. Feeling healthy and in touch with your body can be a bright spot on the horizon, helping you work your way back from low and lonely times. The social function of exercise cannot be overstated. Joining active groups can put you in contact with other people who share your interests. The companionship of a walking partner or a tennis friend can be a lifeline, adding a dimension of hope and playfulness to any life. One 68-year-old woman, when asked about the social aspect of her daily running, replied, "I look forward every day to being with my friends. I couldn't exist without them. They're great!"

Physical Changes

We've listed on the next page the normal changes that you may encounter with aging. Of course, you may not experience every one of these changes; aging varies with the individual and is affected by genetic and environmental factors. The timing of these changes is also difficult to specify because it varies from person to person.

Sometimes these normal changes of aging affect how we function in the world. They limit us in new ways, and we find ourselves wishing we could do the things we were once able to do. Do you find, for instance, that kneeling in the garden is not as easy or as comfortable as it once was? Do you tire more easily? Are you limiting social functions because of urinary incontinence? These changes can be not only frustrating but also wearing on your mental and emotional well-being. Physical limitations can lead to isolation, stress, and feelings of depression, loss, or confusion.

Masking the grief that is sometimes associated with aging can lead to alcoholism or other addictive behaviors. The following story by Virginia tells us how depression around the time of her menopause was affecting her health:

> I was depressed for what seemed years around my menopause. I coped by "numbing out" with alcohol, resulting in my not being there for my kids. I felt unhealthy, fatigued, headachy, and out of shape. With help from friends and therapy, I first tackled my physical well-being. Feeling better, with my self-esteem higher, I was then able to uncover the areas I really needed to work on in therapy. Eventually, I learned to manage my depression and opt for healthy changes in my life.

System Changes Due to Aging

Integumentary (skin)
Lines and wrinkles
Thinning and dryness

Musculoskeletal
Loss of flexibility of joints
Loss of bone density

Endocrine
Decrease in hormones
Decrease in basal metabolism

Sensory
Decreased sight
Progressive hearing loss
Loss of taste sensation
Decreased sense of smell
Decreased ability to distinguish hot or cold

Neurological
Slowing down of reaction time
Changing sleep patterns
Diminished short-term memory

Gastrointestinal
Slowing down of peristalsis/digestion
Decreased ability to absorb and use minerals, nutrients,
    and vitamins

Genitourinary
Decreased muscle tone
Decreased bladder capacity
Thinning and drying of the vaginal walls

Cardiovascular
Increase in size of the heart
Thickening of the valves and blood vessels
Decrease in supply of blood to organs and extremities

Our health is obviously tied to our emotional as well as our physical state. By tackling her alcohol problem, Virginia was able to make her way out of the depression. She began by making changes in her diet and her exercise regime that took into account the limits and possibilities of her changing, aging body. Accepting and becoming comfortable with her body was the first step in restoring her lost vitality and self-esteem.

MENOPAUSE

Menopause is a landmark for all women. It is a biological transition that signals the end of reproductive years, and is defined medically as beginning one year after your final menstrual period. When there is no longer enough estrogen and progesterone to build up the lining of your uterus each month, the monthly flow stops. This change in hormone production is a normal part of the aging process. Menopause can also be brought on surgically by removing the ovaries (bilateral oophorectomy) and, usually, the uterus (hysterectomy).

Not all health-care providers see menopause in the same light. Some subscribe to a "disease model" of menopause based on the thinking that the menopausal woman is estrogen deficient. This is seen as a departure from the "normal," or reproductive phase, of a woman's life. In this framework, menopause is a diagnosed condition, recognized by laboratory tests and doctor's examinations. Robert A. Wilson, in his 1966 book *Feminine Forever*, made explicit the concept of menopause as disease and likened a woman's future without estrogen to a sort of living decay, "in a negative state: dependent, vapid, unfortunate, unseeing, and without vigor."

Wilson's viewpoint is in direct contrast to those who look at menopause as a natural event. In this framework, menopause is neither a disorder nor a departure from the norm. Rather, menopause is a perfectly healthy part of being a woman. As you might imagine, we subscribe to this school of thought. Below you'll find a list of the more common signs to help you recognize your own menopause, as well as some techniques that have helped other women we know.

Signs of Menopause and Ways to Be More Comfortable

In a study begun in 1991, in which Melpomene conducted in-depth interviews with 40 women, the most common sign of menopause reported was hot flushes/flashes, which were reported by 70 percent of the women. Twenty-five to thirty percent of the women reported unusually heavy menstrual flow, irritability, mood swings, and depression.

Twelve percent experienced more painful intercourse. Only 7.5 percent had cold sweats, and 5 percent reported no changes other than an end to menstrual bleeding. While the average number of symptoms reported in this group was 2.5, the range was wide. Women who experience a large number of symptoms, as well as those who experience only one but at a level that significantly alters their lifestyle, would probably benefit from the knowledge that this is not unusual.

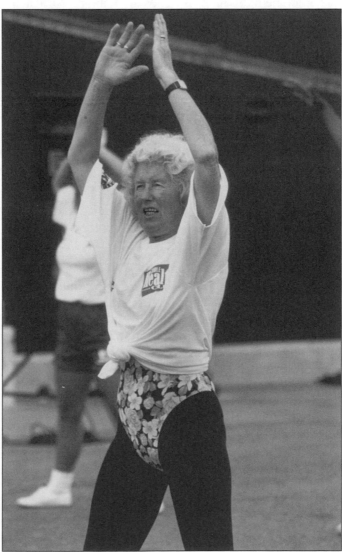

Physical activity during menopause can help you adjust mentally and physically to the changes in your body.

It's important to be good to yourself when your body is undergoing so many changes. A diet high in fresh vegetables, fruit, beans, and whole grains, and low in red meats and saturated fats may bring relief from many of these complaints. Exercising during this time will likely not only boost your mental well-being but also strengthen bone, tone your muscles, and improve circulation, digestion, and elimination. In the Melpomene study, physically active women were more likely to say that their health was "better" or "much better" than most. They also said physical activity helps maintain an appropriate weight for age and height. These facts might encourage more women to consider a physically active lifestyle.

Menstrual Irregularity and Cessation of Menstruation

The period of change is gradual, often starting when a woman is in her mid- to late forties and lasting 5-7 years. Periods may stop abruptly or become irregular or occasionally heavy before tapering off. This heavy bleeding is often the most annoying and worrisome symptom. You will find in talking with your friends or looking at your mother's history of menopause that each individual's experience is unique.

Hot Flashes

Nurse and researcher Ann Voda describes a hot flash as a sudden sensation of heat or a warm feeling. Other sensations include tingling, throbbing, a "rush of blood," light-headedness, chills, and the feeling of suffocation. While most women can expect some form of hot flashes during menopause, the frequency and the length of years in which they are experienced vary widely from person to person. The "triggers" for hot flashes also vary. The common denominator is that hot flashes can be very uncomfortable.

Below are suggestions that may help in alleviating some of this discomfort:

- Eat slowly, and avoid hot liquids (especially coffee and tea), alcohol, and spicy foods.
- Drink ice water, and use cold compresses on your face.
- Take a cool bath, and splash cool water on your face.
- Cool yourself with a fan.
- Dress in layers so you can peel some off.

Vaginal Changes

As estrogen levels in your body diminish, your vagina may become shorter, narrower, and less elastic. The walls will lose their ability to lubricate, and may cause itching or burning, especially during sexual intercourse. Regular sexual activity, if not too uncomfortable, can help the vaginal walls retain their ability to lubricate, even when they have become thinner. You can also lubricate and/or massage the walls of the vagina and vulva area yourself with the following balms:

- Aloe vera gel
- Vitamin E capsules (puncture and use the oil)
- Commercial products, such as Replens, Gynmoistrin, K-Y Jelly, and Astroglyde

Urinary Changes

The lining of the bladder and urethra may also become thin and dry, causing a higher risk of bladder infections, incontinence, and the need to urinate more often during the night. In some women the muscles in the bladder and urethra become weaker. This muscle weakening may lead to a loss of bladder control known as stress incontinence. For example, you may lose a little urine when you cough, sneeze, or laugh. We recommend Kegel exercises to help you strengthen the muscles that control urine flow. Because these exercises are also good for pregnant women, we've included them in chapter 5, page 212, but as they can significantly benefit women going through the changes of menopause, we encourage you to look them over and try them, if necessary.

HORMONE REPLACEMENT THERAPY

Since menopause is characterized by a decrease in estrogen, doctors began to experiment with estrogen supplements in the 1960s. Estrogen replacement therapy became touted as a veritable fountain of youth, promising to help women prevent wrinkles, maintain a youthful silhouette, and keep their hair luxuriant and shiny while eliminating hot flashes, depression, and uncomfortable sexual activity (due to drying and thinning of the vaginal walls).

The balloon burst in the late 1970s when researchers found that women who took estrogen alone were 6 to 14 times more likely to develop endometrial (uterine) cancer than nonusers. However, as more women began to use hormones, doses have been lowered and progesterone has been added in hopes of imitating more closely the balance of hormones in a natural menstrual cycle. This combination of hormones, called hormone replacement therapy (or HRT), is thought

Pearl Jackson: Age Can't Boss Me!

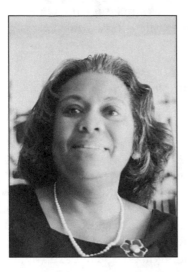

Pearl Mitchell Jackson doesn't like labels, and she doesn't like pigeon holes. She will not be called old, and she will not be forced to fit a stereotype. "What does chronological age have to do with anything?" she asks. "I don't see how your age in years makes a bit of difference. All that really matters is what you've done and how you've done it. I've floated through one life crisis after another. I haven't let a new age bracket frighten me. I floated through menopause. I don't use a lot of new cosmetics and estrogen pills to deal with hitting 35 or 50. It is just another day, not a crisis."

Pearl believes that the way to deal with the aging process is to remain an individual. "You don't have to fit into the cubical that has been set for 50 and 60 and 80 years of age." It's this attitude that keeps Pearl young and helps her to enjoy herself as she takes on yet another one of life's experiences.

"I think of things in a positive way," she says. "Positive thinking is very important in succeeding and moving forward. One of the reasons I am still youthful is that I am able to look at what is good. Even if it is not a beautiful day when I wake up in the morning, I am able to find something beautiful in it. This is very important." Pearl sees herself as "competent and capable." She began her career in the social services and was a volunteer services coordinator for the Ramsay County welfare department for many years. She is now a consultant in international relations and human services doing cross-cultural training.

One of the factors contributing to her positive self-image was growing up in a family involved in multicultural experiences. This allowed her to be comfortable with herself in a variety of milieus, feeling always in place and at home. "My parents taught me very early that when you go someplace, you tell yourself that you belong there. You don't allow yourself to be segregated. I use racism as a stepping stone."

Jackson doesn't deny that she's aging. She says, "Sure, I'm aware of the process, but I never let it become the boss of me. I never let my age tell me what to do."

to prevent the building up of the endometrium (the lining of the uterus) to a precancerous state.

In a 1990 article, "Estrogen Therapy During Menopause and the Treatment of Osteoporosis," researchers Margaret Noyes and Richard Demmler reconfirmed that estrogen is the single most important variable in the prevention of bone loss in postmenopausal women. Estrogen reduces the rate of bone breakdown and allows normal bone building to occur, thus maintaining bone density. Morris Notelovitz is one of several other researchers who have shown that the addition of progestin with estrogen also has a positive effect on bone formation. For this reason, estrogen, alone or in combination with progestin, is often prescribed to help prevent osteoporosis, or thinning of the bones. Most researchers believe that the longer a woman takes estrogen, the more skeletal benefits she derives. Although David Felson and his colleagues, in the 1993 article "The Effect of Postmenopausal Estrogen Therapy on Bone Density in Elderly Women," have shown that a woman needs to take estrogen for a minimum of 7 years to receive a prolonged effect on bone density, most studies have found that estrogen at any point in menopause can slow the rate of bone loss to some extent. Studies have established that use of estrogen early in menopause can, in fact, reduce the risk of fractures by half. However, it is important to remember that protection against bone breakdown lasts only as long as a woman remains on estrogen.

Another important benefit of taking estrogen after menopause is protection against cardiovascular disease. In the United States, heart attack is a leading cause of death among women, but recent studies indicate that hormone replacement therapy can reduce this risk. In fact, many researchers have documented a 50 percent reduction in cardiovascular disease among women taking estrogen alone. Estrogen can protect against heart attack by lowering levels of low-density lipoprotein (LDL, "bad" cholesterol) and increasing levels of high-density lipoprotein (HDL, "good" cholesterol) in the blood. However, with the addition of progestin to estrogen to protect against uterine cancer, researchers Elizabeth Barrett-Connor and Valery Miller in their 1993 article "Estrogen, Lipids, and Heart Disease" have shown that progestin may negatively alter these protective effects for heart disease seen with estrogen alone. For this reason, researchers Donna Session and colleagues, in the *Fertility and Sterility* article "Current Concepts in Estrogen Replacement Therapy in the Menopause," suggest using the lowest dose of progestin in order to receive maximum cardiovascular benefits. However, Barrett-Connor, Miller, and other researchers suggest that this decrease in risk for heart disease may be due to how long a woman takes estrogen, and that the benefits may end once she stops taking the hormone.

Is HRT Right for Me?

To take or not to take HRT, that is the question. The decision about whether or not to begin hormone replacement therapy is one that many menopausal women face. The decision to use HRT depends on your medical history, your menopausal symptoms, and your risk of bone loss and cardiovascular disease. Some women choose not to use hormones because their menopause symptoms are few or because their medical history suggests they are less likely to develop problems related to lower estrogen levels.

Together, you and your health-care provider are the best ones to decide whether HRT is right for you. You should be aware of the wide range of opinion among physicians regarding estrogen replacement. Some consider it a cure-all, while others are hesitant to prescribe it. In many hospitals and clinics, the use of estrogen supplements has become almost automatic. Some physicians are likely to prescribe estrogen for menopausal women without even asking the woman how she feels about it.

> "It is just routine here; when a woman comes in and complains of hot flashes, she is prescribed estrogen. Menopause means estrogen . . . period."
>
> Nurse Practitioner, Midwest Ob-Gyn Clinic

When you visit your doctor, ask her or him to explain what you personally could expect to gain and what you might risk by taking hormones. Make sure all of your questions have been answered before you make your decision. Since individual physicians' opinions about HRT vary, discuss your concerns with other doctors if you do not feel your questions are being addressed. Questions to consider asking your health-care provider include:

- How do you treat menopause?
- How might hormone replacement therapy help me?
- Which forms of hormone replacement therapy do you recommend?
- How will you work with me to determine the best treatment?

The following list describes the risks and benefits of taking HRT. If you are considering the use of hormones, read over this list and write down all your questions and concerns before you go to your doctor.

Considerations for Taking Hormone Replacement Therapy

Benefits
- Eliminates hot flashes
- Reduces vaginal dryness
- Reduces risk of osteoporosis
- Reduces risk of developing heart disease
- May be helpful with insomnia and memory problems

Risks
- Possibly increases risk of developing breast cancer
- Increases risk of gallbladder disease
- Periods and/or cramping may return
- Nausea and vomiting
- Swelling of the ankles, feet, and fingers
- Bloating
- Breast tenderness

Reasons Why HRT May Not Be Recommended
- History of uterine or breast cancer
- Strong family history of estrogen-related cancers (breast, uterus)—should be weighed against family history of heart disease and osteoporosis
- History of thrombotic disorders (formation of blood clots)
- History of uncontrolled or untreated high blood pressure
- Unexplained vaginal bleeding
- History of gallbladder or liver disease

As mentioned previously, estrogen is now most often given in lower dosages and is combined with progesterone. Of the several regimes given, some are accompanied by bleeding and some are not. Each has advantages and disadvantages, but the best method varies according to each woman's needs and preferences. Also, to be effective in the prevention of osteoporosis, estrogen should be combined with a high calcium intake (1,500 milligrams/day) and regular exercise. Some common types and doses of estrogen and progestin treatments are listed in the table on page 260.

Estrogen and Progestin: Types and Doses

Form	Brand Name	Doses (mg)
Estrogens		
Oral	Premarin	.3, .625, 1.25
Tablet	Estrace	1.0, 2.0
	Ogen, Ortho-Est	.625, 1.25
	Estratest	.625, 1.25
Skin patch	Estraderm	.05, .10
Vaginal cream	Estrogen vaginal cream	Varied
Progestins		
Oral	Provera	2.5, 5.0, 10.0
Tablet	Norlutin, Nor-Q-D,	
	Micronor, Aygestin	.35, 5.0
	Ovrette	.075
	Micronized progesterone	100.0
Injectable	Depo-Provera	100.0
	Delalutin, Generic	125.0
	Progesterone	100.0

Hormone replacement is not necessarily for everyone. Jean McCann writes in the February 1993 *Drug Topics* that although 10 to 15 percent of postmenopausal women are on HRT at any given time, the average time on HRT is only 9 months. You need to discuss your specific expectations and needs with your physician and carefully weigh the possible risks you may face. If you decide that you would benefit from hormone replacement, you will want to closely monitor your health while you receive it. Your yearly physical examinations should include a breast examination and possibly a mammogram, a pap smear, and a blood pressure reading. Doctors usually recommend reassessing HRT use on a yearly basis as new information becomes available. It may be beneficial for women to use HRT over prolonged time periods, but information on long-term use is limited.

The latest finding in a series of conflicting studies on the relationship between hormones and breast cancer, reported in "The Use of Estrogens and Progestins and the Risk of Breast Cancer in Postmenopausal Women" by G. Colditz and colleagues in the June 1995 *New England Journal of Medicine*, is that women who continue to use hormone replacement therapy for 5 or more years after menopause are 30 to 40 percent more likely to develop breast cancer than women who have never used menopausal hormones. Previous reports from the same study showed that the risk of developing heart disease was reduced by

50 percent, and deaths from all causes were reduced by 11 percent among current users of postmenopausal estrogen. Therefore, most experts argue that this benefit to the heart more than outweighs any risk of breast cancer.

OSTEOPOROSIS

Fact: Twenty-five million Americans are affected by osteoporosis.

Fact: Eighty percent of those affected by osteoporosis are women.

Fact: Osteoporosis is responsible for 1.5 million hip, wrist, vertebral, and other site fractures annually.

Fact: It is estimated that one out of every two women over age 65 has had an osteoporosis-related fracture.

Fact: White women 60 years of age or older have at least twice the incidence of fractures as African American women. However, one out of five African American women are at risk of developing osteoporosis.

Fact: While osteoporosis is often thought of as an older person's disease, it can strike at any age.

Facts reprinted from National Osteoporosis Foundation.

Osteoporosis, characterized in some women by the dowager's hump, is a major health problem in the United States. From *osteo* meaning "bones," and *porosis* meaning "full of holes," this age-related disorder is characterized by decreased bone mass with increased susceptibility to fractures.

As cited in the National Osteoporosis Foundation 1995 publication "A Status Report on Osteoporosis: The Challenge to Midlife and Older Women," bone mass in women reaches its peak sometime in the early thirties, and remains relatively constant until menopause (or, in some cases, hysterectomy). Then, as estrogen levels drop, the bones begin to lose mass. Osteoporosis, and disabling fractures, can result. During the first 5-7 years after menopause, women can lose from 2 to 5 percent of bone mass each year. After that, the annual rate of loss slows to about 1 percent.

To understand how we lose bone mass, it helps to know something about the bone building and remodeling that goes on in our bodies. Our bones are not static—they are constantly breaking down and rebuilding, usually in a balance that keeps them strong. Estrogen,

Composition of Normal and Osteoporotic Bone

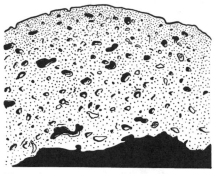

Normal

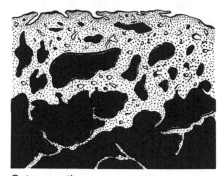

Osteoporotic

calcium, and exercise play major roles in this remodeling process. Weight-bearing exercise and calcium help to actually build bone mass, while estrogen slows the process of bone breakdown. When any of these are in low supply, breakdown can start to outpace buildup, leading to weakened, porous bones, a condition known as osteoporosis.

When bones are thin and full of holes, they become brittle. A minor fall or something as simple as bending over to make a bed can cause a woman with osteoporosis to break a bone or compress her spinal vertebrae. Osteoporosis-related fractures can affect any bone in the body. A 50-year-old Caucasian woman has a 50 percent chance of a fracture sometime in her remaining years, and when over 65, the incidence of hip fracture rises dramatically with age. Of the 1.5 million fractures related to osteoporosis in the U.S. each year, 15 percent are wrist, 25 percent are hip, and 40 percent are spinal. Wrist and hip fractures will happen to one out of six women in the course of a lifetime, and spinal fractures will affect one out of every three women.

Besides bone breakage, the most common structural change associated with osteoporosis is the dowager's hump, a permanent spinal deformity that can cause a woman to lose at least 15 percent of her height, caused by the collapse of vertebrae. Therefore, a woman who has been 5 feet, 4 inches, could lose up to 9 inches by the time she reaches eighty. About 40 percent of all women will have at least one wedge-shaped compression of spinal vertebrae by the time they reach eighty. One woman writes:

> Two years ago my mother, who is 82, fractured her hip after a fall. The physicians weren't sure if she fell and broke her hip or if the hip gave way first. They said she has osteoporosis. I always thought women become "stooped over" because of the burdens

they'd carried for years . . . I've just turned 60, and I noticed that I've lost over an inch in height . . . What is my risk for a hip fracture? Will I have osteoporosis, since my mother has been diagnosed with it?"

Who Is at Risk for Osteoporosis?

As women watch their mothers growing shorter each year, they wonder whether they themselves are at risk for osteoporosis. As you can see from the list shown here, there are definite risk factors that are not under our control: family history, ancestry, being female, and premature menopause. Other factors that put us at risk for osteoporosis are under our control. These mainly include lifestyle habits: level of physical activity, calcium intake, cigarette smoking, and alcohol and caffeine use.

Risk Factors of Osteoporosis

Risk Factors Not Under an Individual's Control
- Premature menopause (natural or surgical)
- Nulliparity (no history of childbirth)
- Family history of osteoporosis
- Northern European ancestry
- Slender body build, fair skin, blond or reddish hair
- Being female
- Associated medical conditions that can independently result in accelerated bone loss—e.g., gastrectomy, anorexia, bulimia, diabetes, kidney or liver disease

Other Risk Factors
- Low level of physical activity
- Low level of calcium intake
- Lifestyle habits: smoking, caffeine, and alcohol use
- Inadequate fluoride level in the water supply
- Being confined indoors
- Ingestion of drugs: anticonvulsants, corticosteroids, antacids containing aluminum (inhibit absorption of calcium) and diuretics (increase the excretion of calcium)

How Is Osteoporosis Detected?

The symptoms of osteoporosis are fractures, the dowager's hump, and the loss of height. There are presently no laboratory tests on the market that will tell you whether you are at risk or whether you already have mild osteoporosis. A small biotechnology company has developed a urine test to measure bone loss, and it is hoped that this test will be available soon. Ordinary x-rays don't clearly detect osteoporosis until 30 percent of bone mineralization is already lost. Certain techniques can measure smaller amounts of bone loss, but these are best used if you are in the high-risk category, or if you are facing a decision about estrogen use. Morris Notelovitz in "Osteoporosis: Screening, Prevention, and Management," 1993, and C.C. Johnston, Jr., and colleagues in an earlier study (1991), cited approximate costs of the procedures, which are listed here. In our experience, these costs may vary by region and specific diagnostic center.

Procedures for Detecting Osteoporosis		
Technique	**Cost**	**Sites Measured**
Single photon	$75-$150	Wrist, heel
Dual photon	$150-$300	Spine, hip, total body
Dual x-ray	$150-$200	Spine, hip, total body
CT scan	$150-$300	Spine

Radiation exposure is relatively low in these scanning techniques, but since radiation poses cancer risk, many women are hesitant to have scans unless they are really necessary. The Scientific Advisory Board of the National Osteoporosis Foundation believes that general screening of all menopausal women is not necessary, but has recommended four situations in which bone mass measurement is indicated:

- Estrogen-deficient women, in order to make decisions about hormone replacement therapy
- Women in whom other diagnostic procedures indicate spinal abnormalities
- Women receiving long-term glucocorticoid (steroid) medicines
- Women with primary hyperthyroidism

From "A Status Report on Osteoporosis: The Challenge to Midlife and Older Women," OWL 1994 & 1995.

We agree that not all women are candidates for routine osteoporosis screening. However, as tests become more sophisticated and are better able to help physicians make treatment decisions, more women may decide that this is an important test to request. You should also note that insurance coverage of bone mass measurement is sporadic. Only about half of private insurance policies cover these tests for diagnostic purposes, and Medicare is inconsistent in its coverage of bone mass measurements.

You'll probably do more for your health by understanding the risk factors and incorporating preventive measures into your lifestyle. If the risk factors listed in this section suggest that you are susceptible to osteoporosis, it is important to consider both prevention and treatment options. Calcium, estrogen, and exercise all have been shown to be important in maintaining bone mass. The various options are discussed below.

Calcium and Osteoporosis

It has been more than a decade since speakers at the National Institute of Health Conference on Osteoporosis first recommended in 1984 that American women significantly increase the amount of calcium in their diets. Since then, hundreds of articles in newspapers and magazines and dozens of television talk shows have focused on osteoporosis and on the role of calcium in preventing brittle bones. As soon as osteoporosis became a household word, marketing departments across the country got busy. Suddenly, a variety of foods from orange juice to cereal were being fortified with calcium. Advertisers played up the calcium content of familiar products such as Tums, which is now perhaps better known as a calcium supplement than as an antacid.

The media focus on calcium is somewhat misleading, however, because calcium alone will not prevent osteoporosis. Estrogen and exercise are also key players in this complex condition. Yet, a high calcium intake may be beneficial for what is called age-related bone loss. Age-related bone loss occurs 10 to 15 years after menopause and therefore is not related to estrogen deficiency. Researchers believe that this bone loss occurs, in part, because the gastrointestinal tract becomes less efficient at absorbing calcium as we get older. This problem is often compounded when women do not take in enough calcium. Studies have shown that an adequate calcium intake can reduce the rate of this age-related bone loss in elderly people.

Are You Getting Enough Calcium?

A 1994 document issued by the National Institute of Health (NIH) recommends a daily calcium intake of between 1,000 and 1,500 milligrams for postmenopausal women. This is a significant increase from the former RDA of 800 milligrams which was based on younger people's needs. The question is not only how much calcium you need but also how your body is using the calcium you consume. Some studies have suggested that premenopausal women also should be consuming 1,000-1,500 milligrams of calcium daily to prevent bone loss. Are you getting enough in your diet? Review the sources of calcium listed below. Chances are you are not consuming enough calcium. Mary Darling and James Johanning, in their 1994 article "Calcium Intakes of Melpomene's Osteoporosis Study Participants," report that only 23 percent of the total participants consumed more than 1,000 milligrams of calcium daily. In order to reach the recommended intake, the women would have had to either eat more calcium-rich foods or take supplements.

Calcium Sources

Milk (2%)—1 cup (300 mg)
Semisoft cheese—1 ounce (200 mg)
Hard cheese—1 ounce (300 mg)
Creamed cottage cheese—1 cup (150 mg)
Yogurt (plain)—1 cup (300 mg)
Grated Parmesan cheese—2 tablespoons
    (150 mg)
Vanilla ice cream—1 cup (170 mg)
Frozen yogurt—1 cup (200 mg)
Cheese sauce—1/2 cup (150 mg)
Cream of tomato soup—1-3/4 cup (300 mg)
Pizza—2 slices (350 mg)
Hot cereal—1 cup (100 mg)
Pancakes—3 (milk added) (150 mg)
Custard pie—1 slice (150 mg)
Almonds, dried—1/3 cup (100 mg)
Broccoli—1 cup (150 mg)
Greens (kale, Swiss chard, collard)—1 cup (300 mg)
Red salmon (canned with bones and oil)—4 ounces
    (250 mg)
Sardines (canned with bones and oil)—2-1/4 ounces
    (350 mg)
Shrimp—4 ounces (150 mg)

Calcium Supplements

While calcium in food is probably more readily absorbed (thus making it the best choice), some women with lactose intolerance will find it difficult to consume the recommended amount because they lack an enzyme that helps to digest lactose-containing foods, such as dairy products. Tablets are available without prescription (Lactaid, Dairy Ease) that contain the missing enzyme. Lactose-free milk is also on the market. Melpomene finds that many women decide to use supplements to make up the difference. The next decision is which kind of calcium supplement to take.

Calcium comes in four basic forms, each of which contains different amounts of usable calcium (see the table below).

Since calcium carbonate has only 40 percent usable calcium, you'd get only 40 milligrams of calcium from a 100-milligram tablet. Calcium gluconate gives you even less; you'd have to quadruple the dosage to wind up with the same amount of calcium you'd get if you took calcium carbonate.

To make sure you are getting what you need, look for one of two things:

1. The percentage of the USRDA. For example, "Each tablet contains 25 percent of USRDA calcium, 250 mg," or
2. The amount of usable or elemental calcium. For example, "Each tablet contains 500 mg of calcium carbonate, which provides 200 mg elemental (usable) calcium."

At Melpomene, we recommend that women take calcium carbonate, which not only provides the most usable calcium but is also generally the least expensive. Calcium carbonate should be taken with a meal to maximize absorption. We also caution women to avoid dolomite and bone meal, which are often contaminated by heavy metals such as lead.

Calcium Supplements

Type of Supplement	Amount of Usable (Elemental) Calcium
Calcium carbonate	40%
Calcium citrate	24%
Calcium lactate	13%
Calcium gluconate	9-10%

Although supplements can be a good way to make sure you've gotten your calcium for the day, they are not without their problems. The more common complaints about supplements include:

1. Large pill size. The pills are large because calcium is a bulky mineral. Alternatives include taking more pills of a smaller dosage, or using chewable tablets or powdered formulas. Be sure to space them out over the day and take with meals in order to enhance absorption. (See the warning that follows about factors that influence calcium absorption and excretion.)

2. High doses may cause constipation or gas. You might be able to avoid gas by increasing your intake slowly over a couple of weeks. If you are still affected, try switching to another brand of supplement.

3. Kidney stones. There is no evidence that calcium alone will cause the formation of kidney stones. Most people can tolerate up to 2,000 milligrams a day without adverse effects. However, if you have a family history of kidney stones, or a predisposition to their formation, consult with your physician before you start taking supplements.

The Best Approach for Preventing Osteoporosis

Besides dietary calcium and supplements, other factors enhance bone building, including estrogen and exercise. Research suggests that a three-pronged program of estrogen therapy, exercise, and calcium seems to offer the best protection against osteoporosis.

Increasing calcium through diet or by taking supplements is only part of the story, however. Other components of your diet or lifestyle may actually be blocking calcium absorption or causing you to excrete it quickly. A good nutritional program of prevention, therefore, stresses: (1) calcium intake, either in natural form, from supplements, or from a combination of the two, and (2) avoiding factors that adversely affect calcium absorption or excretion. See the listing on next page of what influences calcium absorption and excretion.

You don't have to eliminate any of these foods from your diet. In fact, fiber is essential and should not be eliminated. Oat bran is also helpful in reducing cholesterol levels in your blood. If your calcium intake is borderline, these foods should not be eaten at the same meal as the food you depend on for calcium.

Exercise and Osteoporosis

Many researchers have pointed to the importance of physical activity to maintain bone mass. Physical activity is just as important for bone health

Factors That Influence Calcium Absorption

Increase Absorption

Vitamin D—Vitamin D increases calcium absorption from the intestine and reabsorption from the kidneys. A dosage of 400 milligrams a day is recommended. Note, however, that an excess of this vitamin is not only toxic but also causes bone loss.

Fluoride—Fluoridated water promotes calcium retention and bone formation.

Interfere With Absorption

Protein—Red meat is high in phosphorous, a nutrient that prevents calcium absorption. Too much protein also can increase calcium excretion.

Sodium—The more sodium we eat, the more calcium we excrete.

Caffeine and Alcohol—Caffeine and alcohol act as diuretics and increase the loss of calcium through the urine. Alcohol also interferes with calcium absorption.

Phyates—Foods containing phyates may also make calcium unavailable for absorption; examples include oatmeal and bran.

Oxalates—Foods containing oxalic acid in combination with calcium interfere with absorption. These include spinach, rhubarb, sorrel, parsley, and beet greens. Vary these in your diet, and do not use them as a main source of calcium.

Fiber—Fiber interferes with absorption by combining with calcium in the intestine and by increasing the rate at which food is passed through the intestinal tract.

as it is for muscle strength. How does exercise build bones? The two primary mechanical forces applied to bone are muscular contraction and the pull of gravity, and both are responsible for bone rebuilding. If either of these two forces is eliminated, bone mineral content starts to drop. For example, if you are on bedrest, without any weight-bearing or contraction-type exercise, your muscles will atrophy and your bones will lose density. Morris Notelovitz, in a 1993 research article in *Fertility and Sterility*, has suggested that increased bone mass also depends on the type of exercise you do. Women who engage in weight-bearing exercise such as walking, running, or tennis have been shown to have greater bone density than women who participate in non-weight-bearing exercise such as swimming or gardening. However, researcher Susan Bloomfield and colleagues in a 1993 *American Journal of Physical Medicine and Rehabilitation* article report that participating in non-weight-bearing exercise is more likely to increase bone mass than remaining inactive. Weight training has also been deemed to be effective in preventing bone loss in menopausal women, as reported by Leslie Pruitt and other researchers in the *Journal of Bone and Mineral Research*, 1992. Bernard Gutin and M.J. Kasper, in the article "Can Vigorous Exercise Play a Role in Osteoporosis Prevention?," surmise that the combination of weight-bearing exercise with strength training may be the optimal method of preventing bone loss. Here at Melpomene we have been interested in the role of physical activity in preventing osteoporosis since we opened our doors in 1982. The next section details our ongoing work in this area.

Melpomene Osteoporosis Study

In 1982, Melpomene Institute began an ongoing osteoporosis study to answer questions about the relationship between long-term physical activity and bone density. The study group included 111 female subjects, then aged 46 to 80. Fifty-four of the subjects were classified as physically active, while the other 57 were in the physically inactive group. The participants in those two groups were further sorted into six activity levels, based on exercise frequency, intensity, and duration.

Each of the women in our study completed a 12-page questionnaire which included general health history, menstrual history, menopausal history, physical activity patterns, and lifestyle patterns. One hundred and seven subjects completed a 3-day diet log which was then analyzed with a computerized nutritional program. One hundred women underwent computerized tomography (CT) scans of the lumbar spine.

Our goal in this study was to provide factual information that would encourage women to incorporate good nutrition and exercise into their lifestyle. The underlying hypothesis was that women who have engaged in physical activity throughout their lives will have significantly denser bones (more bone mass) than their peers who did not engage in physical activity.

Indeed, this turned out to be true. The average bone density of the physically active women was 25.6 percent higher than that of the

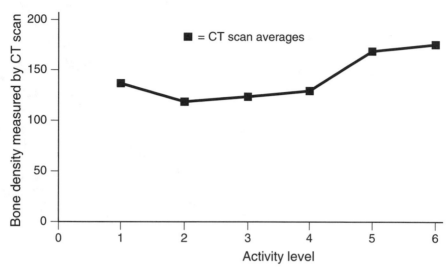

Activity Related to Bone Density

y-axis: Bone density measured by CT scan (0, 50, 100, 150, 200)

■ = CT scan averages

x-axis: Activity level (0, 1, 2, 3, 4, 5, 6)

women in the low-activity groups. Many studies besides our own confirm the finding that exercise does increase bone density and/or decrease significant bone loss in the postmenopausal woman. The results as reproduced here chart how bone density declined with the age of our subjects.

We've continued to measure this group of women periodically over the past 13 years. We have recently measured their bone mass for the third time and soon will be able to report the findings of this study.

Exercises for the Prevention and Management of Osteoporosis

Women with osteoporosis are most likely to fracture a bone in the upper arm at the shoulder, the forearm at the wrist, or the thighbone at the hip and spine. Only the hip and spine can be strengthened by weight-bearing exercises such as walking or running; the arms must be stressed with other specific exercises. The following exercises and guidelines will help you target the areas that need strengthening. Correct posture is also highlighted because it too can prevent certain types of fractures in porous bones.

Material on pages 271-276 is adapted from Brodigan, 1989.

Bone Density Related to Age—Measured by CT Scan

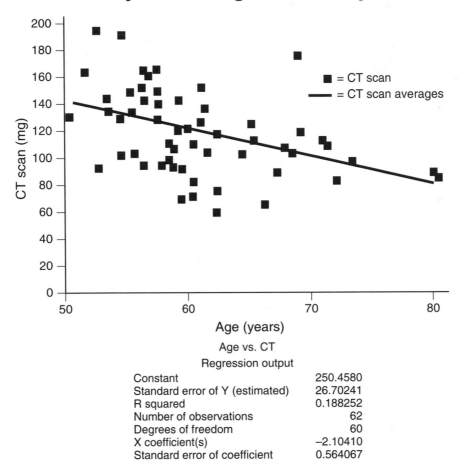

Age vs. CT
Regression output

Constant	250.4580
Standard error of Y (estimated)	26.70241
R squared	0.188252
Number of observations	62
Degrees of freedom	60
X coefficient(s)	–2.10410
Standard error of coefficient	0.564067

Posture Correction.   Sit straight, and stand tall. Align your head directly over your spine. The trunk and limbs should be aligned over your base of support, which is your feet and the space in between. If you lean too far away from your base, you will become unstable, and muscles may become strained. Maintain the natural curve of your low back at all times. Do not lock your knees.

Posture Improvement: Standing and Sitting.   Stand tall, with your hands behind your head. Pinch your shoulder blades together, and press your palms against the back of your head. Resist the forward movement by contracting your neck muscles also. Slowly contract and hold for 5 seconds, while breathing normally. Release slowly. Besides improving rounded shoulders and back, these exercises may also be

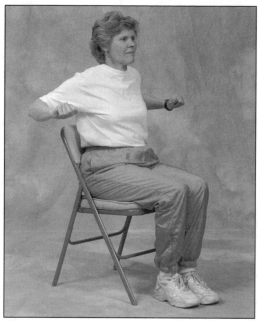

Posture improvement, sitting—hold for 5 seconds.

used to avoid or lessen pain from existing osteoporotic spinal fractures. Sitting or lying positions are better in this case. When sitting, try slowly to press your elbows toward the back. Sit up straight, and hold this position for 5 seconds.

Back Lying.   With your arms perpendicular to your trunk, bend your elbows to 90 degrees and press them into the floor. Hold for 5 seconds, then relax.

Hip and Spine

Specific exercises for the hip and spine should be:

- upright (standing);
- weight-bearing;
- endurance (aerobic) activities, such as walking or mild jogging;
- muscle strengthening, such as isometric abdominal contractions and back extensions; and
- performed for 30 minutes, three or four times per week.

Endurance Activity.   Begin continuous walking with 10 minutes a day. Gradually increase to 30 minutes a day. Always warm up first and use static stretches before and after the activity. Be sure to wear cushioned, low-heeled walking or jogging shoes. Your legs, hip, and spine benefit from working against gravity.

Isometric Abdominal Contraction.   Lie on your back, with your lower back pressed against the floor, and bend your knees to 90 degrees. Tuck your chin to your chest, and contract your abdominal muscles. Hold this position (while breathing normally) for 10 seconds. If osteoporosis is present, avoid rolling your shoulders off the floor; attempt to keep the spine straight and pressed into the floor. Strong abdominal muscles protect the back against strain.

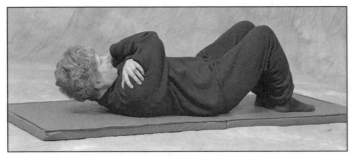

Isometric abdominal contraction. Remember—do not hold.

Back Extension.   Begin on all fours. With back flat, lift one leg so that the heel is level with the buttocks, but no higher. Contract the buttocks and thigh, and hold the position for 10 seconds. When your balance improves, lift the opposite arm simultaneously with the straight leg. Strengthens the back, buttocks, and hamstrings (back of the thigh).

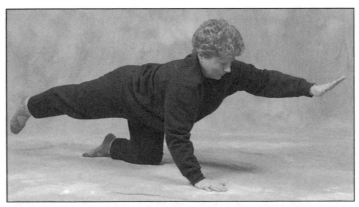

Back extension—hold this position for 10 seconds.

Upper Body

Exercises for the upper body should include:

- weight loading (tension, torsion, compression, bending); and
- resistance exercise with a resistance stretch band. This improves rounded shoulders and back by strengthening supporting muscles.

Resistance stretch bands, such as Thera-Band, often can be purchased from the rehabilitation/physical therapy department at your hospital. You will need about one yard in length. The red band is low resistance; black is the highest resistance.

Tensile Loading. Hang from a bar or pull on a doorknob for 10 seconds. Do not perform this exercise if you have a wrist, elbow, or shoulder injury.

Torsion Loading. With a partner, bend elbows and grasp each other's wrists in the position shown. Attempt to twist your arms in opposite directions against your partner's resistance. Or, grasp a doorknob, and twist your wrist. Hold at maximum resistance for 5 seconds, then reverse direction.

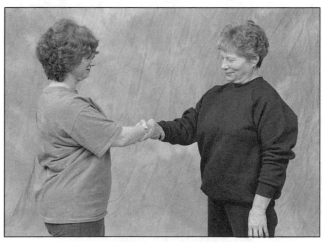

Torsion loading—twist while your partner resists.

Compressive Loading: Sitting Push-Ups. Sitting in a chair with your feet flat on the floor, grasp the edge of the chair seat. Straighten your elbows (but do not lock them) to raise yourself one-half inch off the chair. Hold your weight on your hands for 10 seconds, while breathing normally. Slowly bend your elbows to lower yourself. Try it with the hands in different positions: fingers pointing down, front, or back. Avoid straining or holding your breath (this may be difficult to do, but try your best).

Compressive Loading/Bending.   Begin on hands and knees with the back flat. Contract the abdominal muscles and buttocks to avoid a sagging back. Slowly bend your elbows to 90 degrees (if you can). Let your neck be a natural extension of your spine; do not hang your head. Push up by straightening your elbows. Try one arm alone, and use your fingertips. Or, place your hands in a different supporting position: with arms crossed, with hands wider apart than shoulders, or "creep" hands forward and back while bending the elbows.

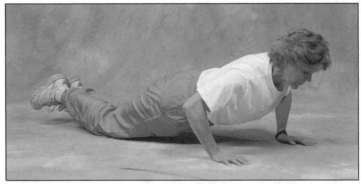

Compressive loading/bending—try to keep your nose beyond an imaginary line between your fingertips.

Resistance/External Rotation.   Grasping a Thera-Band, keep your elbows pressed against your waist and slowly open the forearms outward. Benefits shoulders and rounded back.

Resistance/Horizontal Abduction.   Grasping a Thera-Band, begin with arms straight in front, about chest height. Slowly open your arms to the side. Do not lock your elbows or fling your arms apart. Improves rounded shoulders and back.

EXERCISE AND THE OLDER WOMAN

Here are some of the comments we received from participants in the Melpomene Osteoporosis study:

". . . to be active in life is to be physically involved with life . . . since retirement, I've had more time to be physically active . . . I am more aware of the benefits of exercise."

"I started running when I was 54. I quit smoking after 30 years. I'm now 60, and running is easier now than it has ever been. Exercise has increased my energy level and gives me a sense of well-being."

"I notice a restless feeling after a couple of days of no exercise."

Even though the prevention of bone loss is a major concern of aging women, it is rarely the only motivating force for exercise. Physical activity and fitness have many benefits at all ages. Besides denser bones, exercise offers a sense of accomplishment and well-being, camaraderie, and a feeling of joy. Physically, exercise offers:

- Increased work capacity; more energy
- Lower resting and exercising heart rates
- Lower blood pressure
- Stronger, better-toned muscles
- Flexible joints and ligaments

Older adults gain all the same benefits of physical activity as younger people, but the experience of starting and sticking with a program can often be different. From our work with both active and inactive older women, we offer you the following food for thought.

Should Older Women Exercise?

"I am a 50-year-old woman who has been running for fitness and pleasure for the past 7 years. Approaching menopause as I am, I am beginning to be concerned about various health issues. I find that the medical community has no experience with women who are as active as I am at my age. My health-care provider thinks I shouldn't be running at all. I can't believe that it is all that bad, so I keep on."

A lot of menopausal women come to us with these same concerns. While having a physically active lifestyle is no guarantee that a woman will experience a trouble-free menopause, physical activity helps reduce stress, and helps you to maintain an appropriate weight for your age and height. Besides the influence physical activity has on osteoporosis, as we described earlier, researcher Steven N. Blair and colleagues in a 1992 article, "How Much Physical Activity Is Good for Health?," has shown that a physically active lifestyle is associated with better health and longevity. It also contributes to a reduced risk of cardiovascular disease and adult onset diabetes and possibly lowers the risk of some cancers. While regular vigorous exercise is still recommended for those who want to maintain their health and prevent disease, recent research has shown that light and moderate exercise can also help to improve general physical and mental well-being. In the absence of major illness, no evidence of harm exists. We believe that a regular exercise regime of any kind can only improve an older woman's quality of life.

Results from Melpomene's 1993 research study on menopause suggest that women who are physically active are more likely to report that they feel they are in better health than others their age. Physically active women are also more likely to be able to maintain an appropriate weight for their height and age.

In our osteoporosis study described earlier, we also found that women who were physically active tend to have a more positive perception of "self" than women who were physically inactive. Though the self-perceptions of lower-activity women were not high on the scale, these respondents did report that they were "satisfied" with their appearance and with their lower energy and activity levels. This is not surprising when you consider what has been traditionally deemed appropriate behavior for postmenopausal women. It concerned us, however, that the inactive women in our study were not in good physical shape compared with the active group. The sedentary women reported more sleep problems, less energy, and more muscular aches and pains than the physically active women. Even though most of these women claimed to be "satisfied" with themselves, 20 to 40 percent expressed a desire for change.

What Factors Influence Exercise?

Older women's reasons for exercising (or not exercising) have been an ongoing research interest at Melpomene. We've wanted to know more than just how often and how intensely postmenopausal women are physically active; we've wanted to know why they did it, or why they didn't.

Here's what some women from our studies have had to say about what motivates them to exercise:

"Positive factors affecting my activity? The support and encouragement of my adult children, the availability of facilities, owning a stationary bike for winter and foul weather, the incentive

Factors Influencing Exercise

Motivators
- Previous participation in sports and physical education classes in secondary school and college
- Knowledge of the benefits of activity
- Support and involvement of family and friends in physical activity
- Positive attitudes toward physical activity
- Interest in personal health and fitness
- Habit of regular physical activity

Inhibitors
- Being overweight
- Being a cigarette smoker
- Being too far away from exercise facilities
- Having too little time to participate
- Bad weather

of upcoming runs or cross-country ski races, and personal goals. Bad weather and 'other interests' keep me from my workouts at times."

Connie, age 55

"To maintain motivation to exercise, I've found a partner . . ."

Helga, age 68

Essential to motivation are the feelings of success and reward. All the positive factors may be in place, but unless you have the motivation to get up and get out there time and again, your success will be short-lived. Rewards are excellent reinforcers of behavior. An example is going out to breakfast with your exercise partner or getting yourself new walking shoes. Physical activity should above all be fun: a chance to socialize, wear comfortable clothes and shoes, and do something physical for a change. Don't overdo; walk with purpose, through a park, or to your favorite neighbor's garden. Exercise is more likely to be enjoyable if it is not overly taxing or intense.

If you are an older woman who is just becoming physically active, you may be a pioneer in your community. All of us need to show, by our example, that exercise is both appropriate and healthful for older

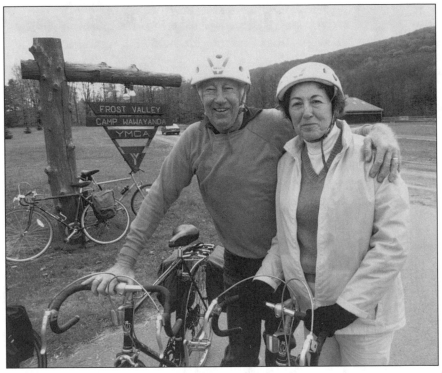

© CLEO Photography

Increase your motivation to be active by exercising with a partner.

women. Of course, we need to paint a realistic picture as well, and be truthful with women who are just staring to become active. Some of the problems that may challenge these women are:

- Lack of support of family and friends

    "My friends and relatives warned that I'll ruin my joints and my bladder will sag from all this running. This puzzles me because I feel so much better when I run."

- Being regarded as old and infantile

    "My family may not want to believe it, but I can make my own decisions. I know what is good for me."

- Having to alter or modify exercise patterns due to the normal aging process

    "Arthritis finally got the best of my daily walking routine. I miss the time with my friends, but we get together for coffee or tea at the Y where I've taken up swimming . . . much easier on my hips, and I still feel active and healthy."

These are difficult areas to confront. Often, as with other parts of the normal aging process, you have no control over the events that limit your ability to maintain exercise patterns. Your ability to accept the changes and make modifications (without losing your enthusiasm) will make all the difference.

Some Tips for Enjoyable Exercise

Whether you exercise on your own, with a partner, or with a group and leader, the warm-up and cool-down are important components in a safe and positive exercise experience. You can warm up by stretching or by doing the activity itself at a low intensity for the first few minutes. The cool-down period after exercise brings the cardiovascular system to a recovery state slowly and helps prevent soreness. Cool-down may include a slow walk, a low-intensity version of the activity, or a series of stretches.

The clothing in which you exercise should be loose for freedom of movement (e.g., an oversized T-shirt), yet supportive where needed (e.g., athletic bras and cushioned socks). There are many new products on the market designed specifically for women. Don't think you're too old to wear shorts in public! Shoes should also be well cushioned and offer good arch and heel support with a nonskid sole.

Older people need to use caution when exercising in hot conditions to avoid the dangers of rapid dehydration and heatstroke. Dehydration can be avoided by routinely drinking eight glasses of water per day, and drinking plenty of water during and after exercise to replace lost fluids. Generally, if you follow this schedule of water replacement, the commercial electrolyte replacements will not be necessary. However, if you are experiencing severe cramps in the legs, arms, or stomach after strenuous physical activity at high temperatures, these may be symptoms of excessive loss of sodium and occasionally potassium and magnesium. The cramping can often be relieved by eating foods or drinking fluids containing sodium chloride. In this case you may wish to try one of the commercially available products, such as Gatorade or another sport drink.

As you age, you should also use caution when exercising in the cold because of the tendency toward vasoconstriction—meaning the small blood vessels constrict, making the heart work harder to maintain the body's heat. Exposed areas such as the fingers, toes, ears, and head must be covered to prevent frostbite. Cover your head to avoid losing heat. The ideal activities in cold weather are those that cause you to generate your own body heat, such as running or cross-country skiing.

Reasons to Stop Physical Activity

- Dizziness
- Chest pain
- Shortness of breath or difficulty catching your breath
- Nausea
- Staggering or persistent unsteadiness
- Mental confusion
- Pallor around the lips
- Profuse sweating along with heart palpitations
- Sharp headache

You should also know about other cautions during physical activity. The table above lists some warning signs that should tell you to stop exercising. Consult your physician or fitness instructor before resuming your usual activities.

What are good forms of exercise? Walking, jogging, cross-country skiing, tennis, bicycling, dancing, bowling, low-impact aerobics, calisthenics, and weight lifting are all good types of exercise for older women. You can maintain a reasonable level of fitness by engaging in an aerobic activity for at least 30 minutes three to four times per week. Even though it is not weight-bearing, swimming is considered a good form of exercise for older women. Because it puts almost no stress on the body, swimming may be a good choice for someone who is arthritic or who has developed osteoporosis.

Walking is another all-round good physical activity that puts very little stress on the body. Walking is weight-bearing and thus helps to lessen the loss of bone mass that leads to osteoporosis. If you are interested in walking, try the following:

1. Start with 10 minutes of easy walking at least three times a week.
2. Gradually walk farther and more often until you are able to walk comfortably for 30 to 40 minutes daily.
3. If you want to increase your cardiovascular endurance, pick up your pace to a walk-jog or add a few hills to your route.
4. Walk heel first in order to minimize strain on the joints.

5. Wear good walking shoes, and dress appropriately for the weather.
6. Listen to your body. Slow down or decrease your distance if you experience persistent fatigue or shortness of breath.

A LAST WORD

We are all aging. For too long, women have dreaded this part of their lives, feeling perhaps that they will have to give up control of their health and well-being when their bodies begin to age. On the contrary, we've described many ways we can enhance our later years, beginning with a lifelong commitment to exercise and good nutrition. In fact, at Melpomene, our research has shown that older women are less stressed and happier in their lives than younger women. In a 1994 study by Judy Mahle Lutter and Kathy Grumstrup about menopausal women, post-menopausal women were found to have more time for exercise and were more likely to believe that their health, happiness, and sense of control were much better than women in other stages of menopause. The end of menopause, for many women, signals the beginning of a new stage of life. There's a great sense of power and confidence when you know enough about your changing body to be able to make informed decisions and keep yourself healthy. With this knowledge, we can take the time to embrace our older selves, reflect upon where we've been, and wonder where our journey may lead us.

References

Chapter 1:
How Far We've Come: A Historical Look at Women and Exercise

Works Cited

Clarke, M.D., and H. Edward. *Sex in Education, or a Fair Chance for the Girls.* Boston: R. Osgood, 1873.

Drinkwater, B.L., ed. *Female Endurance Athletes.* Champaign, IL: Human Kinetics, 1986.

Ehrenreich, B., and D. English. *For Her Own Good: 150 Years of the Experts' Advice to Women.* New York: Doubleday, 1978.

Howell, R. *Her Story in Sport: A Historical Anthology of Women in Sports.* West Point, NY: Leisure Press, 1982.

Yeager, K.K., R. Agostini, A. Nattiv, and B. Drinkwater. *Medicine and Science in Sports and Exercise* 93: 2507, 1993.

Additional References

ACOG Technical Bulletin 189. *Exercise During Pregnancy and the Post Partum Period,* February, 1994.

Boutilier, M.A., and L. SanGiovanni. *The Sporting Woman.* Champaign, IL. Human Kinetics, 1983.

Dyer, K.F. *Challenging the Men: Women in Sport.* St. Lucia, Queensland, Australia: University of Queensland Press, 1982.

Gerber, E.W., J. Felshin, P. Berlin, and W. Wyrick. *The American Women in Sport.* Philippines: Addison-Wesley Publishing Company, 1974.

Howe, J.W., ed. *Sex and Education.* Boston: Roberts Bros., 1874.

Jaffee, L. "Ten Years of Melpomene Membership." *Melpomene Journal,* 11(1) Spring, 35-38, 1992.

Kaplan, J. *Women and Sports.* New York: Avon Books, 1979.

Metheney, E. *Connotations of Movement in Sport and Dance.* Dubuque, IA: Brown, 1965.

Miller Brewing Company. *The Miller Lite Report on American Attitudes Towards Sports.* Milwaukee, WI: Miller Brewing Company, 1983.

Terwilligar, C., "Getting It Straight: How Homophobia Hurts Women in Sports." *Melpomene Journal* 14(1), 5-8, 1995.

Background Information

Title IX—For a summary of provisions and history see *Title IX and Gender Equity* compiled by Karen M. Smith, Assistant Athletic Director, University of Minnesota—Twin Cities.
Women's Intercollegiate Athletics
516 15th Avenue S.E.
Room 250, Bierman Field Athletic Building
Minneapolis, MN 55455

Title IX Information Pack
Women's Sports Foundation
Eisenhower Park
East Meadow, NY 11554

Chapter 2:
What Do You See In Your Mirror?

Works Cited

Bailey, W. *Women and Their Fat.* Covert Bailey Newsletter. 2-3, 1982.

Bennet, N., and J. Gurin. "The Dieter's Dilemma" in *Eating Less and Weighing More.* NY: Basic Books, 1982.

Blackman, S., T. Mertz, and R.D. Singer. "Social Perception of Caloric Value," *Perceptual and Motor Skills*, (55): 535-540, 1982.

Brown Harris, L. *Breast Cancer: A Handbook.* Melpomene Institute, St. Paul, MN, 1992.

Brownell, K. "Obesity: Understanding and Treating a Serious, Prevalent and Refractory Disorder." *Journal of Consulting and Clinical Psychology*, 50(6): 820-840, 1982.

Burk, J., S. Zelen, and E. Terino. "More Than Skin Deep: A Self-Consistency Approach to the Psychology of Cosmetic Surgery." *Plastic and Reconstructive Surgery.* 76(2): 270-280, 1985.

Casper, R.C., and D. Offer. "Weight and Dieting Concerns in Adolescents: Fashion or Symptom?" *Pediatrics* 86(3): 384-390, 1990.

Czajka-Narins, D., and E. Parham. "Fear of Fat: Attitudes Toward Obesity: The Thinning of America." *Nutrition Today*, 26-32, 1990.

Desmond, S.M., J.H. Price, C. Hallinan, and D. Smith. "Black and White Adolescents' Perceptions of Their Weight." *Journal of School Health*, 59(8): 353-358, 1989.

Dyrenforth, S., O. Wooley, and S. Wooley. "A Woman's Body in a Man's World: A Review of Findings on Body Image and Weight Control." In J.R. Kaplan (ed.), *A Woman's Conflict.* London: Prentice-Hall, 31-57, 1980.

Eigner, J. *Body Image and Self-Esteem.* Melpomene Report, 8-12, 1986.

Fallon, A., and P. Rozin. "Sex Differences in Perception of Desirable Body Shape." *Journal of Abnormal Psychology*, 94(1): 102-105, 1985.

Friedman, J., et al. *The Obesity Gene.* The New York Times, A14, 1994.

Gortmaker, S., A. Must, J. Perrin, A. Sobol, and W. Dietz. "Social and Economic Consequences of Overweight in Adolescence and Young Adulthood." *The New England Journal of Medicine*, 329: 1008-1012, 1993.

Howkins, M.A. "Your Weight, Your Health." *Glamour Magazine*, January, 1993.

Jaffee, L., and J.M. Lutter. "Adolescent Girls: Factors Influencing Low and High Body Image." *Melpomene Journal*, 14(2): 14-22, 1994.

Johnson, C. "Raising Largely Positive Kids." *Obesity and Health.* 7(6): 114-115, 1993.

Koff, E., and J. Rierdan. "Perceptions of Weight and Attitudes Toward Eating in Early Adolescent Girls." *Journal of Adolescent Health.* 12: 307-312, 1991.

Lutter, J.M., K. Grumstrup. "Physical Activity and Weight in Menopausal Years: The Melpomene/*Self* Magazine Study." *Melpomene Journal*, 13(1): 17-23, 1984.

Lyons, P., and A. Ansfield. "Body Image and Large Women." *Melpomene Journal*, 7(1): 6-9, 1987.

Lyons, P., and D. Burgard. *Great Shape: The First Exercise Guide for Large Women.* New York: Arbor House, 1988.

Manson, J., M. Stampfer, C. Hennekens, and W. Willett. "Body Weight and Longevity: A reassessment." *Journal of the American Medical Association*, 257(3): 353-358, 1987.

McBride, L. "Teaching About Body Image: A Technique for Improving Body Satisfaction." *Journal of School Health*, 56(2): 76-77, 1986.

Mendleson, B., and D. White. "Development of Self-Body-Esteem in Overweight Youngsters." *Developmental Psychology*, 21(1): 90-96, 1985.

Miller, T.B., J.G. Coffman, and R.A. Linke. "Survey on Body Image, Weight, and Diet of College Students. *Journal of the American Dietetic Association*, 77: 561-566, 1980.

Nichter, M., S. Parker, M. Nichter, N. Vuckovic, C. Sims, and C. Ritenbaugh. *Body Image and Weight Concerns Among African American and White Adolescent Females: Differences Which Make a Difference*, 1994.

Novak Johnson, V. "Children's Socialization Into Sports." *Melpomene Journal*, 8(2): 23-26, 1989.

Robinson, J. "Body Image in Women Over Forty." *Melpomene Report*, 2(3): 12-14, 1983.

Serdula, M.K., M.E. Collins, D.F. Williamson, R.F. Anda, E. Pamuk, and T.E. Byers. "Weight Control Practices of U.S. Adolescents and Adults. *Annals of Internal Medicine*, 119(7) (part 2), 1993.

Stunkard, A.J., T. Sorenson, C. Hanis, T. Teasdale, R. Chakraborty, W. Schull, and F. Schulsinger. "An Adoption Study: Human Obesity." *The New England Journal of Medicine*, 314(4): 193-198, 1986.

Stunkard, A.J., T. Foch, and H. Zdenek. "A Twin Study of Human Obesity." *Journal of the American Medical Association*, 256: 51-54, 1986.

Warviek, P., R. Toft, and J. Garrow. "Individual Differences in Energy Expenditure." In G.A. Gray (ed.), *Recent Advances in Obesity Research*, vol. 2. London: Newman, 1978.

Willet, W., J. Manson, M. Stampfer, et al. "Weight, Weight Change, and Coronary Heart Disease in Women." *Weight and Coronary Heart Disease*, 273(6): 461-465, 1995.

Additional References

Bell, C., and S. Kirkpatrick. "Body Image of Anorexic, Obese, and Normal Females. *Journal of Clinical Psychology*, 42(3): 431-439, 1986.

Connors, M., and C. Johnson. "Epidemiology of Bulimia and Bulimic Behaviors." *Addictive Behaviors*, 12: 165-179, 1987.

Dahlkoetter, J., E. Callahan, and J. Linton. "Obesity and the Unbalanced Energy Equation: Exercise Versus Eating Habit Change." *Journal of Consulting and Clinical Psychology*, 47(5): 898-905, 1979.

Eckholm, E. "That Lean and Hungry Look is No Good as We Age, Controversial Research Says." *Saint Paul Pioneer-Press Dispatch*, August 25: IH, 6-7, 1985.

Feldman, W., E. Feldman, and J.T. Goodman. "Culture Versus Biology: Children's Attitudes Toward Thinness and Fatness." *Pediatrics*, 81(2): 190-194, 1988.

Foster, C., J. Lutter, K. Denny, and C. Kimber. "The Melpomene Institute Body Image Study: A Preliminary Report." *Melpomene Report*, 5(1): 3-8, 1986.

Freedman, R. "Reflections on Beauty as it Relates to Health in Adolescent Females." In S. Golub (ed.), *Health Care of the Female Adolescent*. NY: Haworth Press, pp. 29-45, 1984.

Janelli, L. "Body Image in Older Adults: A Review of the Literature." *Rehabilitation Nursing*, 11(4): 6-8, 1986.

National Institutes of Health. *Technology Assessment Conference Statement: Methods for Voluntary Weight Loss and Control*, 1-29. March 30-April 1, 1992.

Wilson, T. "Assessing Treatment Outcome in Bulimia Nervosa: A Methodological Note." *International Journal of Eating Disorders*, 6(3): 339-348, 1987.

Zurek, L. "Melpomene Research Update." *Melpomene Report.*, 6(1): 18, 1987.

Chapter 3:
How to Get Moving!

Works Cited

American College of Sports Medicine. *Guidelines for Exercise Testing and Prescription*. 3rd ed. Philadelphia: Lea & Febiger, 1991.

Jaffee, L. "Ten Years of Melpomene Membership." *Melpomene* 11, no. 1 (1992): 35-38.

Jaffee, L., and J.M. Lutter. "A Change in Attitudes?" *Melpomene* 10, no. 2 (1991): 11-16.

Additional References

Albohm, M. *Health Care and the Female Athlete.* North Palm Beach, FL: The Athletic Institute, 1981.

Alexander, L.L., and J.H. LaRosa. *New Dimensions in Women's Health*. Boston: Jones & Barlett, 1994.

Anderson, B. *Stretching*. Bolinas, CA: Shelter Publications, 1980.

Bernstein, L., et al. "Prospects for the Primary Prevention of Breast Cancer." *American Journal of Epidemiology* 135, no. 2 (1992): 142-152.

Fait, H., and J. Dunn. *Special Physical Education: Adapted, Individualized, Developmental*. 5th ed. Dubuque, IA: William C. Brown, 1984.

Glover, B., and J. Shepherd. *The Family Fitness Handbook*. New York: Penguin, 1989.

Golding, L.A., C.R. Meyers, and W. Sinning. *Y's Way to Physical Fitness*. 3rd. ed. Champaign, IL: Leisure Press, 1989.

Harris, D., and B. Harris. *The Athlete's Guide to Sports Psychology: Mental Skills for Physical People*. New York: Leisure Press, 1984.

Iknoian, T. "Making Strides." *Women's Sport and Fitness* 16, no. 2 (1994): 55-57.

Johnson, J. "Don't Worry, Be Healthy." *NewsSmith* 9, no. 3 (1994): 12.

Lutter, J.M. "A Question of Age." *Melpomene* 11, no. 1 (1992): 28-34.

McArdle, W., et al. *Essentials of Exercise Physiology*. Malvern, PA: Lea & Febiger, 1994.

Melpomene Institute. *Fitness Walking Guidebook*. St. Paul, MN: Melpomene Institute, 1991.

Meyers, C. *Walking*. New York: Random House, 1992.

Mood, D., et al. *Sports and Recreational Activities*. 10th ed. St. Louis: Mosby-Year Book, 1991.

Ralston, J. *Walking for the Health of It*. Washington, DC: AARP, 1986.

Rippe, J., MD, and Ann Ward, PhD. *The Rockport Walking Program*. New York: Prentice Hall, 1986.

Ritter, M.A., and M.J. Albohm. *Your Injury*. Indianapolis: Benchmark, 1987.

Shangold, M. "Why You Should Exercise." *A Drug Therapy Guide for Women* (January 1986): 83-86.

Sharkey, B.J. *Physiology of Fitness*. 2nd ed. Champaign, IL: Leisure Press, 1984.

Sharp, D. "The Quitter's Exercise Plan." *Health* (June 1994): 68-76.

Shephard, R.J. "Readiness for Physical Activity." *Physical Activity and Fitness Research Digest* 1, no. 5 (1994): 1-8.

U.S. Department of Health and Human Services/Public Health Service. "Public Health Focus: Physical Activity and the Prevention of Coronary Heart Disease." *Morbidity and Mortality Weekly Report* 42, no. 35 (1993): 669-72.

Westcot, W. *Strength Fitness: Physiological Principles and Training Techniques*. 3rd ed. Dubuque, IA: William C. Brown, 1991.

Wilmore, J., and D. Costill. *Physiology of Sport and Exercise*. Champaign, IL: Human Kinetics, 1994.

Wilmore, J. *Sensible Fitness*. 2nd ed. Champaign, IL: Leisure Press, 1986.

Chapter 4:
Menstrual Fact and Fiction

Works Cited

Abraham, G.E. "Nutritional Factors in the Etiology of Premenstrual Tension Syndromes." *Journal of Reproductive Medicine* 28, no. 7 (1983): 446-64.

Aganoff, J., and Boyle, G. "Aerobic Exercise, Mood States, and Menstrual Cycle Symptoms." *Journal of Psychosomatic Research* 38, no. 3 (1994): 183-192.

Baxter-Jones, A., P. Helms, and M. Preece. "Age at Menarche." *Lancet* 343 (February 12, 1994): 423.

Brooks, S.M., C.F. Sanborn, et al. "Diet in Athletic Amenorrhea." *Lancet* (March 10, 1984): 1, no. 8376: 559-60.

Brownell, K.D., et al. *Eating, Body Weight, and Performance in Athletes: Disorders of Modern Society.* Philadelphia: Lea & Febiger, 1992.

Brownell, K.D., et al. "Weight Regulation Practices in Athletes: Analysis of Metabolic and Health Effects." *Medicine and Science in Sports and Exercise* 19, no. 6 (1987): 546-56.

Chauasse, P.H. *Wife and Mother, or, Information for Every Woman.* Philadelphia: H.J. Smith, 1888.

Clark, N. "Athletes with Amenorrhea: Nutrition to the Rescue." *The Physician and Sportsmedicine* 21, no. 4, (1993): 45-48.

Deuster, P.A., et al. "Nutritional Intakes and Status of Highly Trained Amenorrheic and Eumenorrheic Women Runners." *Fertility and Sterility* 46, no. 4 (1986): 636-43.

Drinkwater, B.L., et al. "Bone Mineral Content of Amenorrheic and Eumenorrheic Athletes." *New England Journal of Medicine* 311, no. 5 (1984): 277-81.

Drinkwater, B.L., et al. "Bone Mineral Density After Resumption of Menses in Amenorrheic Athletes." *Journal of the American Medical Association* 256, no. 3 (1986): 380-82.

Drinkwater, B.L., et al. "Menstrual History as a Determinant of Current Bone Density in Young Athletes." *Journal of the American Medical Association* 263, no. 4 (1990): 545-48.

Fort, I., R. DiBrezzo, and J. Forbess. "Activity Level and Menstrual Cycle Function." *Melpomene* 12, no. 2 (1993): 18-20.

Frisch, R.E., and J. W. McArthur. "Menstrual Cycles: Fatness as a Determinant of Minimum Weight for Height Necessary for Their Maintenance of Onset." *Science* 185 (September 13, 1974): 949-951.

Frisch, R.E., and R. Revelle. "Height and Weight at Menarche and a Hypothesis of Menarche." *Archives of Disease in Childhood,* 46 (1971): 695-700.

Plowman, S.A., N.Y. Liu, and C.L. Wells. "Body Composition and Sexual Maturation in Premenarcheal Athletes and Nonathletes." *Medicine and Science in Sports and Exercise* 23, no. 1 (1991): 23-29.

Pirke, K. "Dieting Influences the Menstrual Cycle: Vegetarian Versus Non-vegetarian Diet." *Fertility and Sterility,* 46, no. 6 (1986): 1083-1088.

Prior, J.C., et al. "Conditioning Exercise Decreases Premenstrual Symptoms: A Prospective, Controlled 6-month Trial." *Fertility and Sterility* 47, no. 3 (1987): 402-07.

Ryan, A.J. "Research Studies on the Female Athlete: Gynecological Considerations." *Journal of Physical Education and Recreation* 46, no. 1 (1975): 40-44.

Sanborn, C.F., B.H. Albrecht, and W.W. Wagner. "Athletic Amenorrhea: Lack of Association With Body Fat." *Medicine and Science in Sports and Exercise* 19, no. 3 (1987): 207-12.

Steege, J., and J. Blumenthal. "The Effects of Aerobic Exercise on Premenstrual Symptoms in Middle-Aged Women: A Preliminary Study." *Journal of Psychosomatic Research* 37, no. 2 (1993): 127-133.

Webb, J.L., D.L. Melan, and C.J. Stolz. "Gynecological Survey of American Female Athletes Competing at Montreal Olympic Games." *Journal of Sports Medicine* 19 (1979): 405-12.

Additonal References

Agostini, R. *Medical & Orthopedic Issues of Active and Athletic Women.* Philadelphia: Hanley & Belfus, 1994.

Bell, M., and E. Parsons. "Dysmenorrhea in College Women." *Medical Women's Journal* 38 (1930): 31.

Benson, C. *Handbook of Obstetrics and Gynecology.* Los Altos, CA: Lange Medical Publications, 1980.

Bergfeld, J.A., et al. "Women in Athletics: Five Management Problems." *Patient Care* 21, no. 4 (February 28, 1987): 60-82.

Bergkvist, L., H.O. Adami, et al. "The Risk of Breast Cancer After Estrogen and Estrogen-Progestin Replacement." *New England Journal of Medicine* 321, no. 5 (1989): 293-297.

Boston Women's Health Book Collective. *The New Our Bodies Ourselves.* New York: Touchstone Books, 1992.

Budoff, P.W. *No More Menstrual Cramps and Other Good News.* New York: G.P. Putnam & Sons, 1980.

Bullen, B.A., et al. "Induction of Menstrual Disorders by Strenuous Exercise in Untrained Women." *New England Journal of Medicine* 312, no. 21 (1985): 1349-53.

Cann, C.E., et al. "Decreased Spinal Mineral Content in Amenorrheic Women." *Journal of the American Medical Association* 251, no. 5 (February 3, 1984): 626-32.

Carter, J., and M.J. Verhoef. "Efficacy of Self-Help and Alternative Treatments of Premenstrual Syndrome." *Women's Health Issues* 4, no. 3 (1994): 131-37.

Claessens, A.L., et al. "Growth and Menarcheal Status of Elite Female Gymnasts." *Medicine and Science in Sports and Exercise* 24, no. 7 (1992): 755-63.

Clark, N. "Athletes with Amenorrhea: Nutrition to the Rescue." *The Physician and Sportsmedicine* 21, no. 4, (1993): 45-48.

Costa, M.D., and S.R. Guthrie. *Women and Sport: Interdisciplinary Perspectives.* Champaign, IL: Human Kinetics, 1994.

Fortino, D. "Can Exercise Cure PMS?" *Women's Sports and Fitness* 311, no. 5 (November 1987): 44-47.

Frisch, R.E., et al. "Delayed Menarche and Amenorrhea in Ballet Dancers." *New England Journal of Medicine* 303, no. 1 (1980): 17-18.

Goldin, B.R., et al. "Estrogen Excretion Patterns and Plasma Levels in Vegetarian and Omnivorous Women." *New England Journal of Medicine* 30, no. 25 (1982): 1542-47.

Goodman, L., and A. Gilman. *Pharmacological Basics of Therapeutics.* 8th ed. Riverside, NJ: Pergamon, 1990.

Hensen, A.M., K.F. Immordina, et al. "The Diagnostic Evaluation and Therapy of Secondary Amenorrhea." *Journal of Obstetrics and Gynological Nursing* 13 (1984): 180-84.

Jaffee, L., and J.M. Lutter. "A Change in Attitudes?" *Melpomene* 10, no. 2 (1991): 11-16.

Jones, J. "PMS." *Melpomene Report* 5, no. 1 (1986): 12-17.

Lindberg, J.S., M.R. Powell, M.M. Hunt, et al. "Increased Vertebral Bone Mineral in Response to Reduced Exercise in Amenorrheic Runners." *Western Journal of Medicine* 146, no. 1(January 1987): 39-42.

Lutter, J.M. "Mixed Messages About Osteoporosis in Female Athletes." *Physician and Sportsmedicine* 11, no. 9 (1983): 154-165.

Malina, R., et al. "Menarche in Athletes: A Synthesis and Hypothesis." *Annals of Human Biology* 10, no. 1 (1983): 1-24.

Marcus, R., et al. "Menstrual Function and Bone Mass in Elite Women Distance Runners." *Annals of Internal Medicine* 102 (1983): 158-63.

Merck Manual of Diagnostics. 16th ed. Rahway, NJ: Merck Research Laboratory, 1992.

Monahan, T. "Treating Athletic Amenorrhea: A Matter of Instinct?" *Physician and Sportsmedicine* 15, no. 7 (1987): 184-89.

Mortola, J.F. "A Risk-Benefit Appraisal of Drugs Used in the Management of Premenstrual Syndrome." *Drug Safety* 10, no. 2 (1994): 160-169.

Myburgh, K.H., V.A. Watkin, and T.D. Noakes. "Are Risk Factors for Menstrual Dysfunction Cumulative?" *Physician and Sportsmedicine* 20, no. 4 (1992): 114-25.

Myerson, M., et al. "Resting Metabolic Rate and Energy Balance in Amenorrheic and Eumenorrheic Runners." *Medicine and Science in Sports and Exercise* 23, no. 1 (1991): 15-22.

Nolen, J. "Problems of Menstruation." *Journal of Health, Physical Education, and Recreation* 36 (1965): 65.

O'Brien, P.M.S. "The Premenstrual Syndrome: A Review." *Journal of Reproductive Medicine* 30, no. 2 (1985): 113-25.

Petit, M., and L. Jaffee. "Physical Activity and Contraception." *Melpomene* 10, no. 3 (1991): 18-23.

Prior, J.C. "Endocrine 'Conditioning' With Endurance Training—A Preliminary Review." *Canadian Journal of Applied Sport Science* 7, no. 3 (1982): 148-57.

Prior, J.C. "Luteal Phase Defects and Anovulation: Adaptive Alterations Occurring With Conditioning Exercise." *Seminars in Reproductive Endocrinology*, vol. 3, series 1. Thieme-Stratton, 1985.

Prior, J.C., and Y. Vigna. "The Therapy of Reproductive System Changes Associated With Exercise Training." *The Menstrual Cycle and Physical Activity*. Champaign, IL: Human Kinetics, 1986.

Rebuffe-Scrive, M., et al. "Fat Cell Metabolism in Different Regions in Women." *Journal of Clinical Investigations* 75 (1985): 1973-76.

Ruble, D.M., and J. Brooks-Gunn. "Menstrual Symptoms: A Social Condition Analysis." *Journal of Behavioral Medicine* 2, no. 2 (1979): 171-94.

Scott, E.C., and F.E. Johnston. "Critical Fat, Menarche, and the Maintenance of Menstrual Cycles." *Journal of Adolescent Health Care* 2 (1982): 249-60.

Trussell, J., R.A. Hatcher, et al. "Contraceptive Failures in the United States: An Update." *Studies in Family Planning* 21, no. 1 (1990): 51-54.

Ulrich, C. *Women and Sport—Science and Medicine of Exercise and Sports*. New York: Harper and Brothers, 1960.

Vancouver Women's Health Collective. *PMS: Premenstrual Syndrome, A Self-Help Approach,* 1985.

Warren, M.P. *Clinical Aspects of Menarche: Normal Variations and Common Disorders*. New York: College of Physicians and Surgeons, St. Luke's-Roosevelt Hospital, Columbia University.

Chapter 5:
Keeping Active During Pregnancy

Works Cited

American College of Obstetricians and Gynecologists. *ACOG Home Exercise Programs: Exercise During Pregnancy and the Postnatal Period*. Washington, DC, 1985.

American College of Obstetrics and Gynecology. "Exercise During Pregnancy and the Postpartum Period." *ACOG Technical Bulletin* 189 (1984): 1-5.

Artal, R., et al. "Exercise Prescription in Pregnancy: Weight-Bearing Versus Non-Weight-Bearing Exercise." *American Journal of Obstetrics and Gynecology* 161 (1989): 1464-1469.

Artal, R., R. McMurray, L. Millar, et al. "Recent advances in understanding maternal and fetal responses to exercise." *Journal of the American College of Sports Medicine* 195 (1993):1305-1321.

Bolton, M. "Scuba Diving and Fetal Well-Being." *Undersea Biomedical Research* 7, no. 3 (1980): 183-189.

Clapp, J., and S. Dickstein. "Endurance Exercise and Pregnancy Outcome." *Medicine and Science in Sports and Exercise* 16, no. 6 (1984): 556-562.

Dohrmann, K., and S.A. Lederman. "Weight Gain in Pregnancy." *Journal of Obstetrical, Gynecological, and Neonatal Nursing.* (Nov/Dec, 1986): 446-453.

Franz, M., N. Cooper, L. Mullen, et al. *Gestational Diabetes: Guidelines for a Safe Pregnancy and a Healthy Baby.* Wayzata, MN: International Diabetes Center, 1988.

Jones, R., J. Botti, W. Anderson, et al. "Thermoregulation During Aerobic Exercise in Pregnancy." *Obstetrics and Gynecology* 65, no. 3 (1985): 340-345.

Kulpa, P., B. White, and R. Visschler. "Aerobic Exercise in Pregnancy." *American Journal of Obstetrics and Gynecology* 145, no. 6 (1987): 1395-1403.

Kulpa, P. "Exercise During Pregnancy and Post-Partum." Reprinted from *Medical and Orthopedic Issues of Active and Athletic Women*, edited by Rosemary Agostini, M.D. Philadelphia, PA: Hanley & Belfus, Inc., 1994.

McGrath, M.J., M.F. Mottola, P.J. Ohtake, et al. *Exercise and Sport Sciences Reviews.* Baltimore, MD: Williams & Wilkins, 1989.

Shangold, M., and G. Mirkin. *The Complete Sportsmedicine Book for Women.* NY: Simon & Schuster, 1985.

Veille, J.C., R. Hohimer, K. Burry, et al. "The Effect of Exercise on Uterine Activity in the Last Eight Weeks of Pregnancy." *American Journal of Obstetrics and Gynecology* 151 (1985): 727-730.

Additional References

Berkowitz, G.S., J.L. Kelsey, T.R. Holford, et al. "Physical Activity and the Risk of Spontaneous Preterm Delivery." *Journal of Reproductive Medicine* 28 (1983): 581-588.

Bonen, A., P. Campagna, L. Gilchrist, et al. "Substrate and Endocrine Responses During Exercise at Selected Stages of Pregnancy." *American Physiological Society.* 161 (1992): 134-142.

Chan, G.M. "Human Milk Calcium and Phosphate Levels of Mothers Delivering Term and Pre-Term Infants." *Journal of Pediatrics, Gastroenterology, and Nutrition* 1 (1982): 201-205.

Clapp, J. "A Clinical Approach to Exercise During Pregnancy." In *Clinics in Sports Medicine: The Athletic Woman,* edited by Rosemary Agostini, M.D., W.B. Saunders Co., 1994.

Clapp, J. "The Effects of Maternal Exercise on Early Pregnancy Outcome." *American Journal of Obstetrics and Gynecology* 161 (1989): 1453-1457.

Clapp, J. "Exercise in Pregnancy: A Brief Clinical Review." *Fetal Medicine Review* 2 (1990): 99-101.

Clapp, J. "Pregnancy." *Exercise in Modern Medicine.* Baltimore, MD: Williams & Wilkins (1989): 269-279.

Erdelyi, G. Gynecological Survey of Female Athletes. *Journal of Sports Medicine and Physical Fitness* 12, no. 3 (1962): 174.

Guzman, C.A., and R. Caplan. "Cardiorespiratory Response to Exercise During Pregnancy." *American Journal of Obstetrics and Gynecology* 108 (1970).

Hall, D., and D. Kaufmann. "Effects of Aerobic and Strength Conditioning on Pregnancy Outcome." *American Journal of Obstetrics and Gynecology* 157, no. 5 (1987): 1199-1203.

Hillard, P. "Eating Disorders and Pregnancy." *Parents* (November, 1989): 202-204.

Katz, V.L., R. McMurray, M.J. Berry, et al. "Fetal and Uterine Responses to Immersion and Exercise." *Obstetrics and Gynecology* 72 (1988): 225-230.

Lee, V., and J. Lutter. "Exercise and Pregnancy: Choices, Concerns, and Recommendations." In E. Wilder (ed.), *Obstetric and Gynecologic Physical Therapy.* NY: Churchill Livingstone (1988): 175-198.

Pivarnik, J., W. Lee, and J. Miller. "Physiological and Perceptual Responses to Cycle and Treadmill Exercise During Pregnancy." *Medicine and Science in Sports and Exercise* 23, no. 4 (1990): 470-475.

Rand, C., and D. Willis. "Pregnancy in Bulimic Women." *Obstetrics and Gynecology* 71 (1988): 708-710.

Tafari, N., R.L. Naeye, and A. Gobezie. "Effects of Maternal Undernutrition and Heavy Physical Work During Pregnancy on Birth Weight." *British Journal of Obstetrics and Gynecology* 87 (1980): 222-226.

Uhari, M., and A. Mustonen. "Sauna Habits of Finnish Women During Pregnancy." *British Medical Journal* 1 (1979): 1216.

Wong, S.C., and D.C. McKenzie. "Cardiorespiratory Fitness During Pregnancy and its Effect on Outcome." *International Journal of Sport Medicine* 8 (1987): 79-83.

Chapter 6:
Your Child's Fitness

Works Cited

American Association of University Women. *Shortchanging Girls, Short-changing America.* 1991.

Blair, S. "Are American Children and Youth Fit? The Need for Better Data." *Research Quarterly for Exercise and Sport* 63, no. 2 (1992): 120-23.

Bunker, L.K. "The Role of Play and Motor Skill Development in Building Children's Self-Confidence and Self-Esteem." *Elementary School Journal* 91, no. 5 (1991): 467-71.

Feminist Majority Foundation. "New Report on Gender Gap in Sports Features Scoreboard of Inequities." Arlington, VA, 1995.

Gilligan, C., N. Lyons, and T. Hamner. *Making Connections: The Relational Worlds of Adolescent Girls at the Emma Willard School.* Cambridge, MA: Harvard University Press, 1990.

Hill, G.M. "PASS: Guidelines for K-6 Games and Relays." *Strategies: A Journal for Physical and Sport Educators* 7, no. 3 (1993): 5-8.

International Food Information Council. "Kids Make the Nutritional Grade." Washington, D.C., 1992.

Jaffee, L., and J.M. Lutter. "Adolescent Girls: Factors Influencing Low and High Body Image." *Melpomene* 14, no. 2 (1995): 14-22.

Jaffee, L., and R. Manzer. "Girls' Perspectives: Physical Activity and Self-Esteem." *Melpomene* 11, no. 3 (1992): 14-23.

Jaffee, L., and S. Ricker. "Physical Activity and Self-Esteem in Girls: The Teen Years." *Melpomene* 12, no. 3 (1993): 19-28.

Kolata, G. "A Parents' Guide to Kids' Sports." *New York Times Magazine*, April 26, 1992.

Nelson, M.A. "Development Skills and Children's Sports Participation." *The Physician and Sports Medicine* 19, no. 2 (1991): 67-79.

Novak Johnson, V. "Children's Socialization Into Sport Study." *Melpomene* 7, no. 1 (1988): 13.

Novak Johnson, V. "Children's Sports Socialization Study." *Melpomene* 6, no. 1 (1987): 15-17.

Schlicker, S.A., et al. "The Weight and Fitness Status of United States Children." *Nutrition Reviews* 52, no. 1 (1994): 11-16.

Seefeldt, V., et al. 1992. "Overview of Youth Sports." Commissioned paper by the Carnegie Council on Adolescent Development. Washington, DC, 1992.

Strong, W.B., and J.H. Wilmore. "Unfit Kids: An Office-Based Approach to Physical Fitness." *Contemporary Pediatrics* 5, no. 4 (April 1988): 33-48.

Stucky-Ropp, R., and T. DiLorenzo. "Determinants of Exercise in Children." *Preventive Medicine* 22 (1993): 880-889.

"Survey Says More Kids Putting on Too Many Pounds." *Minneapolis Star Tribune,* October 3, 1995, 7A.

U.S. Department of Health and Human Services, Center for Disease Control. "Youth Risk Behavior Surveillance—United States, 1993." *Morbidity and Mortality Weekly Report* 44 (SS-1) (March 24, 1995).

Weiss, M.R., and L.M. Petlichkoff. "Children's Motivation for Participation in and Withdrawal From Sport: Identifying the Missing Links." *Pediatric Exercise Science* 1 (1989): 195-211.

Yu, V. "Portrayals of Females in Sports Picture Books: An Examination of Children's Picture Books With Sports Themes." *Melpomene* 12, no. 3 (1993): 14-18.

Additional References

American Sport Education Program. *SportParent.* Champaign, IL: Human Kinetics, 1994.

Baranowski, T., et al. "Assessment, Prevalence, and Cardiovascular Benefits of Physical Activity and Fitness in Youth." *Medicine and Science in Sports and Exercise* 24 (6 supp.) (1992): S237-47.

Boutilier, M.A., and L. SanGiovanni (eds.). *The Sporting Woman.* Champaign, IL: Human Kinetics, 1983.

Chrysler Fund-AAU Physical Fitness Program. *Fitness Trends in American Youth: A Ten Year Study 1980-89.* September 14, 1989.

Cooper, K.H. *Kid Fitness.* New York: Bantam, 1991.

Foster, C.D. "Learning to Deal With Success and Failure: Children's Casual Attributions." *Melpomene Report* 2 (May 1983): 11-13.

Gabbard, C.P., and S. Crouse. "Children and Exercise: Myth and Facts." *The Physical Educator* 45, no. 1 (winter 1988): 39-43.

Greendorfer, S.L. "Gender Bias in Theoretical Perspectives: The Case of Female Socialization Into Sport." *Psychology of Women Quarterly* 11 (1987): 327-40.

Helion, J.G., and F.F. Fry. "Modifying Activities for Developmental Appropriateness." *Journal of Physical Education, Recreation, and Dance* 66, no. 7 (1995): 57-59.

Hellstedt, J.C. "Kids, Parents, and Sports: Some Questions and Answers." *The Physician and Sports Medicine* 16, no. 4 (1988): 59-71.

Holland, M. "Fitness for Kids: An Approach That Works." *Melpomene* 7, no. 3 (1988): 22.

McGinnis, M.J. "The Public Health Burden of a Sedentary Lifestyle." *Medicine and Science in Sports and Exercise* 24 (6 supp.) (1992): S196-200.

McKenzie, T.L., et al. "Children's Activity Levels and Lesson Context During Third-Grade Physical Education." *Research Quarterly for Exercise and Sport* 66, no. 3 (1995): 184-93.

McMurray, R.G., et al. "Parental Influences on Childhood Fitness and Activity Patterns." *Research Quarterly for Exercise and Sport* 64, no. 3 (1993): 249-55.

Novak Johnson, V. "Melpomene Research Reports: Children's Socialization Into Sport Study." *Melpomene* 7, no. 2 (1988): 15-20.

Pate, R.R., and J.G. Ross. "The National Children and Youth Fitness Study II: Factors Associated With Health-Related Fitness." *Journal of Physical Education, Recreation, and Dance* (November/December 1987): 45-48.

Quinn, P.B., and B. Strand. "Children and Youth Fitness: Where Are We and Where Are We Going?" *California Alliance for Health, Physical Education, Recreation, and Dance Journal* 56 (1993): 9-12.

Ross, J.G., and G. Gilbert. "The National Children and Youth Fitness Study: A Summary of Findings." *Journal of Physical Education, Recreation, and Dance* 56, no. 1 (November/December 1985): 45-50.

Ross, J.G., and R.R. Pate. "The National Children and Youth Fitness Study II: A Summary of Findings." *Journal of Physical Education, Recreation, and Dance* 58, no. 9 (1987): 51-56.

Rowland, T.W., and P.S. Reedson. "Commentaries: Physical Activity, Fitness, and Health in Children: A Close Look." *Pediatrics* 93, no. 4 (1994): 669-72.

Sallis, J.F., et al. "Determinants of Physical Activity and Interventions in Youth." *Medicine and Science in Sports and Exercise* 24 (6 supp.) (1992): S248-57.

Snyder, E.E., and E. Spreitzer. "Correlates of Sport Participation Among Adolescent Girls." *Research Quarterly* 47 (1976): 804-09.

Tarr, S. "Adapting Equipment for Special Needs." *Strategies* 6, no. 3 (1992): 24-27.

U.S. Department of Health and Human Services, Center for Disease Control. "Vigorous Physical Activity Among High School Students—United States, 1990." *Morbidity and Mortality Weekly Report* 41, no. 3 (January 24, 1992).

Wilcox, R.C. "Promoting Parents as Partners in Physical Education." *The Physical Educator* 45, no. 1 (winter 1988): 19-23.

Wilson Sporting Goods Company and the Women's Sports Foundation. *The Wilson Report: Moms, Dads, Daughters, and Sports*. June 7, 1988.

Chapter 7:
Age and the Active Woman

Works Cited

Barrett-Connor, E., and V. Miller. "Estrogen, Lipids, and Heart Disease." *Clinics in Geriatric Medicine* 9, no. 1 (1993): 57-67.

Blair, S.N., H.W. Kohl, N.F. Gordon, and R.S. Paffenbarger. "How Much Physical Activity Is Good for Health?" *Annual Review of Public Health* 13 (1992): 99-126.

Bloomfield, S.A., N.I. Williams, D.R. Lamb, and R.D. Jackson. "Non-Weightbearing Exercise May Increase Lumbar Spine Mineral Density in Lumbar Spine in Healthy Postmenopausal Women." *American Journal of Physical Medicine and Rehabilitation* 72, no. 4 (1993): 204-209.

Brodigan, D.E. *Melpomene* 8, no. 1 (1989): 22-23.

Colditz, G.A., S.E. Hankinson, D.J. Hunter, W.C. Willett, J.E. Manson, M.J. Stampfer, C. Hennekens, B. Rosner, and F.E. Speizer. "The Use of Estrogens and Progestins and the Risk of Breast Cancer in Post-menopausal Women." *New England Journal of Medicine* 332, no. 24 (1995): 1589-1593.

Darling, M.E., and J.A. Johanning. "Calcium Intakes of Melpomene's Osteoporosis Study Participants. A Comparison of 1982, 1984 and 1990 Food Records." *Melpomene* 13, no. 3 (1994): 20-24.

Felson, D.T., Y. Zhang, M.T. Hannan, D.P. Kiel, P.W.F. Wilson, and J.J. Anderson. "The Effect of Postmenopausal Estrogen Therapy on Bone Density in Elderly Women." *New England Journal of Medicine* 329, no. 16 (1993): 1141-1146.

Gutin, B., and M.J. Kasper. "Can Vigorous Exercise Play a Role in Osteoporosis Prevention?: A Review." *Osteoporosis International* 2 (1992): 55-69.

Johnston, C.C., C.W. Slemenda, and L.J. Melton. "Clinical Use of Bone Densitometry." *New England Journal of Medicine* 324, no. 16 (1991): 1105-09.

Lutter, J.M., M. Betrand, S.W. Strom, and K. Grumstrup. "Menopause and Physical Activity: What Is the Relationship?" *Melpomene* 12, no. 1 (1993): 14-23.

Lutter, J.M., and K. Grumstrup. "Physical Activity and Weight in the Menopausal Years: The Melpomene/*Self* Magazine Study." *Melpomene* 13, no. 1 (1994): 17-23.

McCann, J. "Many Dropouts on Estrogen Replacement—For a Reason." *Drug Topics,* February 8, 1993.

Nabulsi, A.A., A.R. Folsom, A. White, W. Patsch, G. Heiss, K.K. Wu, and M. Szklo. "Association of Hormone-Replacement Therapy With Various Cardiovascular Factors in Menopausal Women." *New England Journal of Medicine* 328, no. 15 (1993): 1069-75.

National Institute of Health. "Optimal Calcium Intake." NIH Consensus Statement 12, no. 4, June 6-8, 1994.

National Osteoporosis Foundation. "Legislative Issue Brief—Bone Mass Measurement. Fast Facts on Osteoporosis. A Status Report On Osteoporosis: The Challenge to Midlife and Older Women." 1995.

Notelovitz, M. "Osteoporosis: Screening, Prevention, and Management." *Fertility and Sterility* 59, no. 4 (1993): 707-25.

Noyes, M.A., and R.W. Demmler. "Estrogen Therapy During Menopause and the Treatment of Osteoporosis." *Primary Care* 17, no. 3 (1990): 647-66.

Pruitt, L.A., R.D. Jackson, R.L. Bartels, and H.J. Lehnhard. "Weight-Training Effects on Bone Mineral Density in Early Postmenopausal Women." *Journal of Bone and Mineral Research* 7, no. 2 (1992): 179-85.

Session, D.R., A.C. Kelly, and R. Jewelewicz. "Current Concepts in Estrogen Replacement Therapy in the Menopause." *Fertility and Sterility* 59, no. 2 (1993): 277-84.

Voda, A.M. "Alterations of the Menstrual Cycle." In P. Komnenich (ed.), *The Menstrual Cycle.* NY: Springer, 1981.

Voda, A.M. "Coping With the Menopausal Hot Flash." *Patient Counsel, Health Education* 2 (1982): 80-83.

Wilson, R.A. *Feminine Forever.* NY: Evans Press, 1966.

Additional References

Bilezikian, J.P. "Major Issues Regarding Estrogen Replacement Therapy in Postmenopausal Women." *Journal of Women's Health* 3, no. 4 (1994): 273-282.

Hazzard, W.R. "Estrogen Replacement and Cardiovascular Disease: Serum Lipids and Blood Pressure Effects." *American Journal of Obstetrics and Gynecology* 161 (1989): 1847-1853.

Isaia, G.C., G. Salamano, M. Mussetta, and G.M. Molinatti. "Vertebral Bone Loss in Menopause." *Experimental Gerontology* 35 (1990): 303-307.

Lobo, R.A. "Cardiovascular Implications of Estrogen Replacement Therapy." *Obstetrics and Gynecology* 75, no. 4 (supp.) (1990): 18S-25S.

Meunier, P.J. "Prevention of Hip Fractures." *American Journal of Medicine* 95 (supp. 5A) (1993): 75S-78S.

Rikli, R.E., and B.G. McManis. "Effects of Exercise on Bone Mineral Content in Postmenopausal Women." *Research Quarterly for Exercise and Sport* 61, no. 3 (1990): 243-49.

Rosenberg, L., J.R. Palmer, and S. Shapiro. "A Case-Control Study of Myocardial Infarction in Relation to Use of Estrogen Supplements." *American Journal of Epidemiology* 137, no. 1 (1993): 54-63.

Stampfer, M.J., and G.A. Colditz. "Estrogen Replacement Therapy and Coronary Heart Disease: A Quantitative Assessment of the Epidemiologic Evidence." *Preventive Medicine* 20 (1991): 47-63.

Wolf, P.H., J.H. Madans, F.F. Ficucane, M. Higgins, and J.C. Kleinman. "Reduction of Cardiovascular Disease—Related Mortality Among Postmenopausal Women Who Use Hormones: Evidence From a National Cohort." *American Journal of Obstetrics and Gynecology* 164 (1991): 489-94.

Other Resources for Older Women

Newsletters

"A Friend Indeed," published by A Friend Indeed Publications, Inc., Box 515, Place du Parc Station, Montreal, Quebec, H2W 2P1, or P.O. Box 1710, Champlain, NY 12919-1710.
$30 for 10 issues.

"Hot Flash," published by the National Action Forum for Midlife and Older Women (NAFOW), P.O. Box 816, Stony Brook, NY 11790-0609.
Free sample issue; $25 for subscription.

"Midlife Woman," published by Midlife Women's Network, 5219 Logan Avenue South, Minneapolis, MN 55419-1019.
$25 for six bimonthly issues.

Brochure

"Hormone Replacement Therapy (HRT): Is It For Me?" by Hanna Cooper and Judy Mahle Lutter. Medical consultants: Susan Cushman, MD, and Patricia Kohls, MD. Available from the Melpomene Institute, 1010 University Avenue, St. Paul, MN 55104.
Price: $2.50

Index

About the Authors

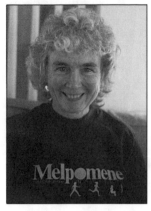

Judy Mahle Lutter is the cofounder and president of the Melpomene Institute for Women's Health Research, America's only organization devoted to health issues affecting physically active women. Judy began running in 1973 at the age of 33. Five years later, she recorded her personal best time of 2:56 at the Boston Marathon and became known around town as an expert on women and running. Recognizing the shortage of research on physical activity and women's health, she began conducting her own studies and in 1982, she and her friend Susan Cushman, MD, formed the Melpomene Institute to help women make informed choices about their own health and lifestyles.

A popular speaker on the topic of physical activity and health for women, Judy is on the advisory board of the Women's Sports Foundation. She has won numerous awards in the health and fitness arena and has been a guest columnist for several fitness publications, including *Women's Sports and Fitness, Runner's World*, and *FootNotes*. She also writes a weekly column for the *St. Paul Pioneer Press*. Judy holds two master's degrees from the University of Minnesota—one in American studies and one in educational psychology. A competitive distance runner, cyclist, and cross-country skier, Judy is a mother of three. She and her husband, Hap, live in St. Paul, Minnesota.

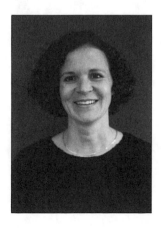

As Melpomene Institute's program coordinator, **Lynn Jaffee** is responsible for organizing and implementing research projects and educational programs. Some of her research projects involve physical activity and body image among adolescent girls, physical activity and women recovering from chemical dependency, health and physical activity patterns of larger women, and amenorrhea and menstrual cycles among athletes.

Lynn speaks to groups around the country and writes numerous articles for the *Melpomene Journal* and other publications on many of the topics she researches. She holds a bachelor's degree in health and human services from Metropolitan State University in St. Paul, Minnesota, and a certificate in health and lifestyle counseling from the St. Mary's campus of the College of St. Catherine in St. Paul. Lynn's hobbies include running, cycling, backpacking, and bird watching. She and her husband, Steven, have two children and live in Hopkins, Minnesota.

You'll Benefit from Joining Melpomene

When you become a member of Melpomene Institute, you become part of an active, caring organization that offers you a number of important benefits. These include a subscription to the *Melpomene Journal*, an authoritative and practical source of new research information, updates, and general interest articles; discounts on Melpomene publications, events, videos, and gift items; and free use of the Resource Center, which holds more than 4,500 articles and research studies. Membership costs $32 a year.

MELPOMENE'S NEWEST OFFERINGS

- **Heroes: Growing Up Female and Strong**
  A 52-minute video, originally aired as a prime time documentary, focuses on the link between self-esteem and physical activity for adolescent girls. Video and curriculum materials: $24.95. Video only: $19.95.

- **Breast Cancer: A Handbook**
  This 122-page, spiral-bound book is a companion for a woman, her family, and friends while she gathers information, learns about her options, and makes decisions about her treatment and self-care as a cancer patient. This handbook, written by Linda Brown Harris, is complete, concise, and handy. $8.95.

- **Of Heroes, Hopes, and Level Playing Fields**
  A collection of insights and observations on physical activity and women. The book selects 40 of Judy Mahle Lutter's *Women in Sports* columns from the St. Paul Pioneer Press. $10.00

For information about membership or products, please contact us:

Melpomene Institute
1010 University Avenue
St. Paul, MN 55104

Phone: 612/642-1951
Fax: 612/642-1871
e-mail: melpomen@webspan.com
web site: http: // www.stpaul.gov/melpomene/

Founded in 1982, Melpomene Institute for Women's Health Research helps women and girls of all ages link physical activity and health through research, publication, and education.

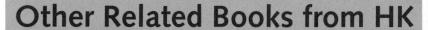
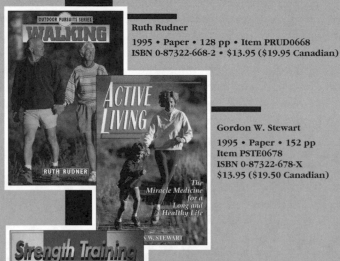
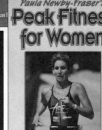